Cholesterol: Facts and Fantasies

Third revised and expanded edition

Judith A. DeCava, CNC, LNC

seleneriverpress
select books on nutrition health

PO Box 270091
Fort Collins, Colorado 80527
866-407-9323
www.seleneriverpress.com
info@seleneriverpress.com

Second expanded edition 2005

Third revised and expanded edition 2015

Cover Design by Stefanie Berganini/WTF Marketing

ISBN 978-1-941277-17-1

Made in the United States of America

Saturated fat and cholesterol in the diet are not the cause of coronary heart disease. That myth is the greatest scientific deception of this century, perhaps any century.

George V. Mann, MD
Professor of Medicine and Biochemistry
Vanderbilt University, 1991

Contents

Cholesterol: Facts and Fantasies

Cholesterol is a necessary part of every cell in the human body and is imperative in virtually all aspects of metabolism. We would die without it.

Cholesterol forms 50% of the nervous system; it is necessary for proper development and growth of the brain and nervous system and serves as a conductor of nerve impulses. Cholesterol helps to form membranes for billions of cells where it regulates the exchange of nutrients and waste products. It is an essential part of bile salts which assist digestion, particularly of fats; without complex food fats, vitamins A,D,E,F and K (fat-soluble vitamins) could not be absorbed. Cholesterol is an important component in hormones produced by the adrenal glands, sex glands (gonads), and pituitary gland. It is needed in the skin to convert sunlight into vitamin D and to provide a barrier in the skin to prevent water or other fluids from inappropriately entering the body. It plays a part in calcium metabolism and bone structure, in heart muscle contraction, and liver function.

A deficiency of cholesterol results in fatigue, obesity, nervous and emotional disturbances, digestive difficulties, impotency or inability to conceive and/or complete a pregnancy, menstrual syndromes and masculine traits in women, effeminate traits in men, blood pressure irregularities, fluid imbalances, nutritional deficits and imbalances, and more.

In 1990, 635,000 Americans died of cardiovascular disease (coronary heart disease and stroke). Cholesterol is one of the major culprits blamed for this 20th century epidemic. Medical experts tell us that high serum (blood) levels of cholesterol cause heart attacks and that it is an accurate indicator of a worsening disease situation leading to heart attack. Diet, we are informed, is a root factor governing cholesterol levels and therefore coronary heart disease.

Yet when persons diagnosed 'sick' with 'high' cholesterol levels change their diets to low fat or low cholesterol, there is usually little or no reduction in cholesterol levels in their blood. Obviously, this tactic does not work.

Russell L. Smith, Ph.D. is the author of the book, *The Cholesterol Conspiracy*, which is derived from his huge scientific publication entitled, *Diet, Blood Cholesterol and Coronary Heart Disease: A Critical Review of the Literature.* Dr. Smith states that, "Both the public and clinical physicians have simultaneously been swamped by an ever-growing tidal wave of exaggerations, distortions and even fabrications of the facts." And he proves it.[1]

Cholesterol and Food

There is only about five ounces of cholesterol in the body; approximately 7% of that (one-third of an ounce) circulates in the blood. Around 80% of cholesterol in the body is produced by the liver; the intestinal wall produces additional amounts and, when necessary, it is synthesized in every cell of the body except nerve cells. The body manufactures between 1,000 mg and 2,000 mg a day – by far the body is the major producer of cholesterol found within it. We are told by the medical establishment to eat only 300 mg or less of cholesterol in foods, yet the body produces four to seven times that amount itself. Obviously, cholesterol is needed and the body knows it. [1]

Studies show that the more cholesterol consumed in food, the less the body produces. If little or no cholesterol is consumed, the more the body tries to produce. In other words, the level of one's blood cholesterol remains virtually constant regardless of whether a little or a lot of cholesterol is eaten.

One case to illustrate the point is an 88-year old man, a retirement-home resident, who has consumed 20 to 30 eggs a day for more than 15 years. The AHA recommends no more than three eggs a week because of their cholesterol content. Still this octogenarian who simply loves soft-boiled eggs, consistently has blood cholesterol levels between 150 to 200. The National Cholesterol Education Program sets levels below 200 as the 'acceptable maximum.' Dr. Fred Kern, Jr. of the University of Colorado School of Medicine, learned about the elderly egg eater and, upon study, became fascinated with him. Said Kern, "I asked, 'How does this man have a normal cholesterol level?'" What Dr. Kern found at work were two efficient biological systems which have been known for many years: the man absorbed only a small amount (18%) of the cholesterol from his intestinal tract, and most of what was absorbed was converted into bile acids.

(Most people normally consume less cholesterol and 50 to 60% is absorbed.) So his body absorbed what was needed, utilized what was absorbed, and excreted the rest; his body retained proper balance. This man has consumed about 5,300 mg of cholesterol a day for 15 years! The AHA says to keep it to 300 mg. Why does this elderly man crave eggs? As Dr. David G. Williams suggested, "It's highly possible his unusual cravings are linked to a specific need for some nutrient found in eggs."

Dr. Antonio Gotto, former resident of the AHA, was asked to comment on the elderly egg lover. He noted that only one-third of all people have an increase in their blood cholesterol levels when they eat extra cholesterol or fat; 65 to 75% of the population may not be negatively affected. This is a startling admission from a staunch promoter of the cholesterol theory! Why do the Gottos of this world try to scare and pressure everyone to limit eggs, meat, and other high-cholesterol foods from the diet? Margaret Flynn, a clinical dietician at the University of Missouri in Columbia, said the elderly man's normal cholesterol is not surprising. "All of the studies we have done showed no effect [on blood cholesterol] of high egg consumption in a normal diet," she said. And as one science journalist remarked, "Many people know of an elderly relative who starts every day with sausage and bacon and two over easy but never has a twinge of heart trouble." As the body can balance cholesterol properly under normal circumstances, eating cholesterol-rich foods will not elevate blood cholesterol, and cholesterol cannot be blamed for heart attacks.[2]

HDL and LDL

Cholesterol and fat travel together in tiny "ships" made of protein. Since cholesterol and fat (triacylglycerols) are both lipids (fats or fatlike substances), the little "ships" are 'lipoproteins.' There are five types of lipoproteins. The cholesterol content of all five lipoproteins is measured when blood is drawn and the sum is the total cholesterol. Recently, two specific lipoproteins have been stressed in the news: HDL (high-density lipoprotein) or so-called "good" cholesterol, and LDL (low-density lipoprotein) or so-called "bad" cholesterol. The cholesterol in both HDL and LDL is exactly the same, so the "good" and "bad" labels seem inappropriate.

HDL contains primarily one type of protein (apolipoprotein A-I or ApoA-I) whereas LDL contains primarily another type of protein (ApoB-100). This protein difference and the fact that HDL particles contain more protein and less fat than the LDL are the bases of calling HDL "good" and LDL "bad." Yet, "the exact precursor-product relationships between the other types of plasma lipoproteins (besides the chylomicrons and VLDL and including HDL and LDL) **are yet to be completely defined, as are the roles of the various protein components...**The role, if any, of high-density lipoprotein (HDL) in transport of lipid-based energy **is yet to be clarified.**"[3] (Emphasis added)

In other words, both HDL and LDL contain the exact same kind of cholesterol and the differences between the two are in the type and amount of protein they contain. It is not known what the roles of the protein components are, and it is not known if HDL plays a part in transporting fats or cholesterol. Nevertheless, the NHLBI/AHA alliance teaches that HDL is "good" because it presumably picks up cholesterol from artery walls and removes it from the blood, and LDL is "bad" since it presumably sticks to blood vessel walls and causes atherosclerosis. This is all entirely speculation!

Persons with low HDL or high LDL are told they are candidates for a heart attack based on this theory. "But reports to the annual meeting of the American Heart Association say not all people with a low HDL level run a high risk of a heart attack. In fact, some people whose HDL level was thought to be alarmingly low turn out to have no more than a normal risk of heart attack.[66]

The research that led to this revelation included the discovery of many "patients with low HDL levels who don't have coronary heart disease," as Dr. H. Bryan Brewer of the NHBLI reported. Their explanation? A particular type of HDL that contains a particle of ApoA-I "seems to provide superior protection against the ravages of heart disease," and, even if HDL levels are low, this particular type of HDL is protective whereas HDL deficient in this protein makes a person a higher risk for heart disease. This is truly amazing since biochemists already knew that the prime factor distinguishing HDL from LDL is HDL's prominent protein ApoA-I! If it's always been there, what has changed?[5]

4

Another confusing report comes from a study which found that people can increase their HDL if they jog or walk while on a low-fat diet. But if they follow a low-fat diet without exercising, they can reduce their level of the "good" HDL, presumably increasing their risk of heart disease. Does this then mean that low-fat dietary recommendations potentially increase heart attack rates?[6]

Further, people on a low-fat diet reduced their "bad" LDL even more if they had small LDL particles in contrast to those people who had large LDL particles. If the chemical makeup and amount of LDL is bad, what difference would size make?[7]

The enzyme, lipoprotein lipase, is reported to remove the fat (triacylclycerol) from very-low-density lipoprotein (VLDL which contains even more fat than LDL) to form smaller and denser lipoproteins that may become LDL particles. Yet a massive increase in blood fat (triacylglycerol) concentrations and low HDL in persons without lipoprotein lipase enzyme - a situation that would be considered dangerous in medical circles – "does not seem to predispose them to atherosclerosis ['clogging' of the arteries]."[8]

Factors That Affect Blood Cholesterol Levels

Genetics is one of the primary determinants of cholesterol levels in the blood. If a group of people all ate the exact same diet, their cholesterol levels would still remain different.

An underactive thyroid (hypothyroidism) is a "classical cause" of high cholesterol levels. Mental stress, work, and standing up can change cholesterol levels temporarily. A person's cholesterol level actually varies throughout the day. Nicotine use, pain, fear, pregnancy, lack of exercise, a number of drugs and medicines (such as male and female hormones, tranquilizers, cortisone products, diuretics, and even alcohol) increase cholesterol levels. Kidney disease, diabetes, hepatitis, and gallbladder obstructions also raise cholesterol. The longer a tourniquet is bound to the arm while blood is being drawn, the higher the cholesterol level.[1]

Blood cholesterol fluctuates constantly and may be entirely different during different seasons of the year. It is often higher during cold weather, though there is no real consistency of the times peaks and troughs occur, depending on the individual and even where he or she lives. Individual variations of up to 30% have been observed. Variations in plasma cholesterol levels are reflected in changes in LDL and HDL as well. There are week-to-week and day-to-day variations.

During one study, cholesterol levels were found to swing from 21% above to 20% below the level measured at the beginning of the trial. Variation of cholesterol level over the period of time of another study averaged about 25%; in fact, 21 of the people in this study had variation of over 50%! Many investigators recommend repeated cholesterol measurements before any assessment can be made of average cholesterol level. Observations of the cholesterol cycles and variations "emphasize the need for caution and deliberation in assessment of risk... Certainly multiple analyses must be completed before risk is assigned and/or treatment initiated or rejected."[10]

Dr. Edward Pinckney, former associate editor of the *Journal of the American Medical Association*, wrote: "The laboratory test for cholesterol is probably the most inaccurate test there is. It is considered medically acceptable for results to be 50 mg off in either direction."[11]

More than one study has shown that normal or low cholesterol is no guarantee of cardiac fitness. In one study, almost half of the patients had total cholesterol levels below 200, the present acceptable 'safe' maximum. Yet, half of this group had coronary artery disease. Of the almost 1,200 who had documented heart disease, one-third had cholesterol levels below 200. Dr. Michael DeBakey, the famous heart surgeon, reports that 30% of patients who have a coronary bypass have 'normal' cholesterol levels.[12]

Since 60% of people in this country normally have cholesterol levels between 200 and 330 (the maximum normal level prior to 1988), and because cholesterol levels normally increase with age, "how can a condition be called hyperlipidaemia [high blood cholesterol] if it occurs in most of the population?"[13]

How the Scam Began

In the early 1900s, experiments were conducted in which rabbits were fed very large amounts of dietary cholesterol every day. Their blood cholesterol rose from a normal of about 100 mg to as much as 2,000 mg. In a short time, a soft plaque-like disease formed on their coronary arteries and other blood vessels. When the cholesterol feeding was stopped, the plaque gradually disappeared. Thus was formulated the theory that dietary cholesterol is the cause of high blood cholesterol and atherosclerosis (the build-up of hard plaque on the inner walls of the arteries feeding blood to the heart muscle). There ensued literally thousands of experiments with millions of animals of all types, even quail. If diet is the cause of coronary heart disease (CHD), why has it been necessary, for about 80 years, to conduct thousands of animal experiments to try to prove it?

Rabbits and other animals do not metabolize (process) cholesterol like humans. While huge amounts of dietary cholesterol raise blood cholesterol in humans only a few milligrams (if that), they raise levels in rabbits many hundreds of milligrams. The type of cholesterol fed to the rabbits in the experiment was a synthetic form easily oxidized when exposed to air. Oxidized products are very toxic. In the normal human diet, foods containing cholesterol naturally contain vitamins and antioxidants which protect the body from toxic oxidation.

Animals which do metabolize cholesterol similar to humans, such as rats and dogs, when fed large amounts of cholesterol, do not develop the atherosclerosis-**like** disease as did the rabbits. In fact, it was eventually found that the atherosclerosis-like disease **could** be caused in a variety of animals with almost any major nutrient — protein, carbohydrates, saturated and polyunsaturated fats – if given too much.

In 1925 it was discovered that dietary cholesterol was not the chief source of blood cholesterol; the body itself manufactures far more.

That atherosclerosis-**like** disease which developed in animals was similar to, but **not** atherosclerosis. The **soft** plaque formed in the arteries of rabbits and other animals was not the same as **hard** plaque found in human atherosclerosis (which does not disappear or even reduce in size when diet is changed). Scientists have **never** been able to produce a hard plaque in animals by feeding them cholesterol for over 80 years. Dr. Mark Altschule called the thousands of animal experiments "worthless." Despite this tremendous difference between animals and humans, it was still assumed that dietary cholesterol was the cause of CHD.

The idea might have died out in the 1950s if it were not for Dr. Ancel Keys, a University of Minnesota physiologist, who proposed (in the early part of the decade) that fat (not dietary cholesterol it-self) was the cause of high blood cholesterol in humans and thus the cause of atherosclerosis. By the late 1950s it was discovered that all fats did not raise blood cholesterol levels. Then it was proposed that saturated fats increased cholesterol, polyunsaturated fats decreased cholesterol, and monounsaturated fats were neutral (although today they are thought to lower cholesterol).

In 1957 a group of AHA members and supporters reviewed all the research literature up to that time; their report to the AHA concluded that the American diet had not changed over the years in ways that could make it the cause of the increase in CHD deaths. Regardless, in 1961, the American Heart Association (AHA) adopted Dr. Keys' unproven theory and he became the cover story in *Time* magazine, elevating him to medical stardom. The 1957 report was rejected.

The AHA made its first dietary recommendations in 1961, coun-seling the public to replace "substantial" amounts of saturated fats with polyunsaturated fats. (Today the AHA recommends low poly-unsaturated-fat diets because research found high polyunsaturated-fat diets – primarily with refined, hydrogenated or partially hydro-genated fats – depress the immune system and promote the growth of cancers.) As a consequence of their recommendations, a measure of fear developed in people's minds about cholesterol and dietary cholesterol.

The well-known Framingham study began in 1948. Some 6,000 men and women were periodically studied, examined, and followed for many years. Around 1960, the first principal report indicated that the higher the blood cholesterol, the higher the tendency for CHD rates. This association was made (between cholesterol and CHD) for the **group** of participants but not for virtually all the separate indi-viduals within the group. The NHLBI and AHA accepted the group results and ignored the individual results.

In 1970 another major report from the Framingham study re-vealed that **no association** could be found between what the people participating ate and either the level of blood cholesterol or eventual development of CHD. This report was never published.

When a US Senate Select Committee on Nutrition and Human Needs convened in 1976 and 1977, the issue of diet and CHD was raised to national prominence. Dr. Robert Levy, Director of NHLBI, provided the primary testimony. Even though he admitted that no scientific evidence existed which showed that CHD could be reduced by diet or by lowering cholesterol, he still urged Congress to recommend the "Prudent Diet" for everyone. Cholesterol was to be limited to 300 mg per day (rather than the typical 500 mg), total fat was to be reduced to 30-35% of total calories (down from the usual 36-37%), and that fat be equally divided among saturated, polyunsaturated, and monounsaturated. The Committee agreed.[1]

The Numbers Game

The NHLBI/AHA alliance has constantly told both the public and physicians that CHD is an epidemic of our century. Heart disease has been the number one killer in the US, true. But 40% of all heart attacks occur in persons whose arteries are not narrowed by atherosclerosis. Atherosclerosis is the 'disease' linked to diet by the alliance. Death statistics lumping all heart attacks together exaggerate the true frequency of deaths involving atherosclerosis.

There was a 21% increase in CHD death rates from 1950 to 1962; this was the 'epidemic.' Yet, death rate due to all heart diseases decreased substantially as the CHD death rate increased. It would be expected that the CHD 'epidemic' would drive all heart disease death rates upwards. The reason for this conflict is, "as physicians increasingly classified deaths due to CHD after 1950, they decreasingly classified deaths due to hypertensive heart disease and endocarditis and other myocardial degeneration." They took from one classification and gave to another – 'robbing Peter to pay Paul.' Really, it was simply changing the classifications of the deaths.[1]

The CHD death rate jumped upwards in 1968 and suddenly downwards in 1979. Still, the all-heart disease death rate trend remained the same. Prior to 1968, hypertensive (high blood pressure) heart disease was classified separately from CHD. In 1968, hypertensive heart disease began to be considered a part of CHD, so CHD appeared to suddenly increase. In 1979, hypertensive heart disease was again classified as separate from CHD, so CHD appeared to suddenly decrease. The all-heart-disease death rate trend never changed through all of this – only the classifications changed.[1]

The CHD rate continued to increase since 1968 in England and Sweden despite the fact that their peoples were doing all the same things that people in the US have done to supposedly decrease CHD.[14]

The recorded CHD death rate peaked in 1962 and then began to decline in 1964. By 1986, it had declined 45% and still continued and continues downward. The alliance claims that the decline is due to changes like following low-fat diets, a reduction in cigarette smoking, and a reduction in blood pressure among Americans. Yet NHLBI's Kannel and Thorn admitted in 1984 that "no one has yet established a convincing fit of trends for any risk factor with cardiovascular mortality trends."[1] As mentioned above, other countries doing the same things did not experience a reduction in CHD rate. There has been no real evidence linking the assumed 'risk factors' (or the reduction of 'risk factors') to CHD deaths.

Technical, medical, and emergency advances since the 1960s have prolonged the lives of persons with CHD. These machines, drugs, and facilities prolong but do not "cure" the disease and actually place the patients at increased risk of dying from many other diseases and non-diseases, especially cancer and accidents. So, even though CHD death rate decreases, it is compensated for by increases in other death rates. Cancer deaths, for instance, have been increasing as fast as CHD deaths have been decreasing.[1] In 1990, 635,000 Americans died of cardiovascular diseases (heart attack, stroke). Cancer killed about 500,000 people.

Additionally, letting the proverbial cat out of the bag, Dr. William Kannel announced in 1989 that data from 30 years of the Framingham study show that all cardiovascular diseases, including CHD and stroke, have **increased** in frequency.[15] The National Centers for Disease Control, in a 1989 press release, revealed that CHD was on the **increase** nationwide.[16] In 1992, the economic cost of cardiovascular disease – doctors, nurses, hospitals, medications, lost work time – totaled $108.9 billion![17] Therefore, while the recorded CHD **death** rate may seem to be decreasing due to improved emergency treatment, the frequency of the **disease** is increasing.

Food and Fat Trends

Cholesterol occurs only in animal foods such as meats, eggs, dairy products, and seafood. It is claimed that increased consumption of animal fats, and thus cholesterol, greatly contributed to the epidemic in cardiovascular disease.

Some 12 studies investigating food consumption since 1909 all showed that animal fat consumption did not increase in this century; it actually decreased about 10%. Total fat did increase by 26% and saturated fat did increase by 10%, but these increases were primarily from vegetable oils and margarines – items that are supposedly helpful in preventing cardiovascular disease! The total increase in vegetable-fat use since 1909 was over 200%![1] "Animal fat consumption has not increased in the past sixty years. The increase in heart attacks has paralleled the increased consumption of margarine, homogenized milk, and other processed foods." The proportion of animal fat in the American diet decreased from 83% in 1910 to 62% in 1972 during the heart attack 'epidemic.'[18]

Saturated fat, the supposed 'bad' fat as in animal fats, occurs in significant amounts in natural vegetable fats too. Saturation of vegetable fats is increased when hydrogenation is performed to make margarine and other solid or semi-solid fats from vegetable oils. For instance, coconut oil (used in many processed foods) is over twice as saturated as pork fat; coconut oil is 95% saturated, pork fat is 40% saturated.[19]

Before 1900, when heart attacks were extremely rare, almost all dietary fats were from animal products; vegetable fats were virtually nonexistent. After his study of food consumption trends, NHLBI's Dr. Harold Kahn admitted that "the increased risk of CHD reported to have occurred over this period is not related to dietary fat changes to a very important degree."[20] If CHD were related to fat, then it would have to be related to vegetable fat!

Cholesterol and Heart Attacks

The blood cholesterol levels for Americans range from below 100 mg to over 1,000 mg, though most levels are between 110 mg and 350 mg; the average is about 220 mg. Cholesterol levels increase with age. Women tend to have lower levels than men under the age of 45 but higher levels than men after age 45. Despite the fact that women have much higher blood cholesterol levels after age 45, it is well known that they have much lower CHD rates.[1]

We are told by the NHLBI/AHA alliance via the media that the higher the blood cholesterol level, the greater the risk of a heart attack.

The Framingham Study was started in 1948 and involved about 6,000 people from Framingham, Massachusetts. One group of persons who consumed large amounts of cholesterol and saturated fat were compared to a group who consumed less cholesterol and saturated fat. This study has now been in progress for over 40 years and there continues to be no difference in coronary heart disease (CHD) between those persons on the "bad" (high cholesterol) diet and those on the "good" (low cholesterol) diet.

Regardless, Dr. William Kannel of the Framingham Study announced that there was a "powerful" relationship between cholesterol and CHD. The figures and graphs used showed CHD "events" (deaths PLUS other CHD incidents) versus blood cholesterol levels ranging from 84 mg to 1124 mg. The intervals of cholesterol levels shown were not all the same; they were: 84 to 204 mg; 205 to 234 mg; 235 to 264 mg; 265 to 294 mg; and 295 to 1124 mg. The middle three intervals had a 30 mg difference. The first interval (84 mg to 204 mg) had a 120 mg difference. The last interval (295 mg to 1124 mg) had a 829 mg difference! This method is not legitimate for making accurate evaluations. Obviously a graph with such intervals would show a sharp upsurge in CHD "events" around the beginning of the last interval. This is a gross distortion of the actual facts! Only about 5% of the entire population has cholesterol levels above 295 mg. These people sometimes have serious diseases such as diabetes and genetic defects that not only elevate cholesterol levels but also promote CHD-like disease.[1] This would also make it seem as if higher cholesterol levels increase CHD, but that is not the case.

An even larger study (362,000 men) published in 1986 was the Multiple Risk Factor Intervention Trial (MRAT). This study was used by the alliance in the National Cholesterol Education Program for setting the "borderline high cholesterol" (200 to 240 mg) and "high cholesterol" (over 240 mg) labels. Going from the lowest to the highest cholesterol levels in all these men, the CHD death rate increased 0.13%–statistically insignificant and trivial! Again, the graphs used by the researchers used unequal intervals in an effort to make the results conform to the preconceived idea (and justify all the time and money spent, no doubt) that the higher the cholesterol, the higher the CHD rate.

These are only two examples of how public statements and arbitrary rules are made which "often do not conform to the scientific data..."[1]

The level of blood cholesterol does not, for the vast majority of people, distinguish between those with or without CHD. "Most people with CHD have low to moderate levels of cholesterol and most people with high levels of cholesterol do not die of CHD. These facts are fully acknowledged in the medical literature."[1]

"For the majority of Americans, cholesterol reduction does not appear to make a major contribution to improving life expectancy," said Dr. William C. Taylor of Beth Israel Hospital, Boston."[21]

Professor emeritus of nutrition at the Harvard Schools of Medicine, Dr. D. Mark Hegsted, admitted: "In the U.S. about one-half of heart attacks apparently occur in individuals with serum cholesterol levels below 240 mgldL."[22]

Columbia University's H. Kaunitz stated: "One study showed that the most severe lesions [of CHD] at autopsy occurred in people who had quite low serum cholesterol values."[23]

"One-half of all heart attacks now occur in people whose serum cholesterol is 225 mg or less," noted Dr. William Castelli.[24] Since the average blood cholesterol level is about 220 mg, this statement means that heart attacks occur equally across all cholesterol levels.

In the large MRFIT study, of the men who died of CHD, "62% had total cholesterol levels less than 240 mg."[25]

It is obvious that the relationship between blood cholesterol level and CHD is extremely weak at best, and nonexistent upon a close look at the scientific data.

Diet and Blood Cholesterol Levels

The cholesterol theory proposes that people who eat a diet high in saturated fats and cholesterol have elevated blood cholesterol and a high rate of coronary heart disease (CHD).

Warren S. Browner, M.D., MPH, and his colleagues at the School of Medicine, University of California at San Francisco, asked: "What If Americans Ate Less Fat?" as the title of a scientific article. Based on the assumptions of restricting fat intake to 30% of calories to reduce heart disease and other diseases such as cancer, that reducing blood cholesterol levels will reduce coronary heart disease death rates, some interesting figures were revealed. If all the 'cholesterolmania' scares were true, there would be only a 2% benefit, equivalent to a three- or four-month increase in life expectancy, and this would apply chiefly to people over age 65. "These results may be disappointing to those who believe that following a healthier [sic] diet will protect them from early death," said Browner.[26]

After consideration of the MRC Epidemiology Unit Caerphilly and Speedwell Studies in the United Kingdom, a Medical research Council panel concluded that the results "provide no basis for altering public health recommendations about diet." The findings of the studies revealed less heart disease in men who drank more milk and used butter rather than polyunsaturated margarine. So the panel could not find a reason to tell people to reduce their milk and butter consumption.[27]

Another study was performed to determine if persons already consuming a low-fat diet would show a change in their blood cholesterol levels by feeding them more cholesterol in their diets (with eggs). The total cholesterol and the LDL and HDL fractions "did not differ significantly."[28]

The findings of the MRC's Epidemiology Unit that milk and butter – "hitherto presented as dietary villains – may be protective has sent shock waves through the ranks of officialdom." Dr. W.W. Yellowless cites the Norwegian cholesterol lowering regimen during the 1950s during which soy margarine replaced butter and soy oil was used extensively. The increase in the use of soy-oil products during the next 20 years was accompanied by a steep and continuing rise in deaths from heart attack (coronary thrombosis). Despite many, many dissidents (prominent physicians and researchers) who have "argued against the theory that coronary heart disease can be prevented by changes in fat consumption," the populace is still advised to reduce saturated fat consumption to 30% and increase polyunsaturated fats."[29]

Seventy young men (18 and 19 years old) were divided into three groups which ate either 3, 7, or 14 eggs a week for five months. These participants had similar cholesterol levels in the beginning and were checked during the study for any changes in total cholesterol, LDL-cholesterol, and HDL-cholesterol levels; triglycerides (neutral blood fats), and their blood-clotting factors. There were no significant changes among the groups. "It seems that egg intake in this range did not influence CHD risk markers in these subjects." In other words, eating eggs (or other cholesterol-containing foods) does not increase risk of heart attack.[30]

In another study, men and women "with moderately-elevated serum cholesterol" were randomly placed in three groups: (1) the control group who ate their usual diet, (2) those placed on a low-fat diet, and (3) those placed on a low-fat, high-fiber diet. All three groups experienced reductions in cholesterol, but the group eating more fiber-rich foods experienced the most significant reduction – a much greater reduction than the low-fat group. The low-fat group and the high-fiber group both ingested the same amount of fat and cholesterol, so fiber-rich foods were not replacing fats in the diet; they were added to the diet. Could it be that the consumption of whole, natural foods (like beans and oats used in this study) which are rich in fiber too, would balance cholesterol and other fat-metabolism factors much more so than a low-fat or low-cholesterol diet?[31]

Walnuts and other nuts have been spurned as high-calorie, high-fat foods. Findings of one study indicate that walnuts lower total cholesterol levels.[32] Palm oil, a maligned tropical oil with a high amount of the dreaded saturated fats, was found to lower cholesterol levels. "Palm oil," said lead researcher Kenneith C. Hayes, "probably doesn't raise cholesterol in individuals with normal cholesterol metabolism."[33]

A "meta-analysis" (a study of many studies) of the effects of dietary cholesterol on blood cholesterol levels resulted in some strained, though revealing, conclusions. People who desire to reduce their blood cholesterol by dietary restrictions would have to reduce their dietary cholesterol to minimal levels (under 100 to 150 mg a day...

the current medical recommendation is 300 mg a day) to observe "modest" blood cholesterol reductions. Persons eating a diet rich in cholesterol would have little if any change in blood cholesterol after adding even large amounts of cholesterol to their diet. In other words, a highly-restrictive diet virtually eliminating all cholesterol foods would result in only a small reduction of blood cholesterol, whereas a diet already rich in cholesterol would not elevate blood cholesterol even if more cholesterol foods were added. Then why make cholesterol lowering changes to the diet at all?[34]

"Nineteen trials conducted over a period of 31 years had failed to show that low-fat, low-cholesterol diets would prevent coronary heart attack."[35]

"The largest part of the general population (perhaps...two-thirds) have the least to gain by lowering cholesterol levels," stated Dr. E.H. Ahrens, Jr., Rockefeller University. Dr. Ahrens maintains, after more than 40 years of research, that there is no scientific evidence to show that the low-fat "Prudent Diet" recommended by the AHA will reduce the risk of CHD.[36]

"Diet does not have a profound influence on plasma cholesterol concentrations in Western populations," explains Maria C. Linder, Ph.D., California State University, Fullerton. Dr. Linder says that a drastic reduction in cholesterol intake generally results in only a small decrease in total blood cholesterol concentrations (10 to 15%). This reduction has been shown to have little effect on risk of CHD or dying from heart disease.[37]

The International Atherosclerosis Project, published in 1968, collected data on 12 subpopulations. No associations were found between the amount of animal fat consumed and the amount of atherosclerosis or between animal fat consumed and the level of blood cholesterol. The study concluded that animal fat was not related to CHD; this conclusion is never mentioned by the alliance.[1]

Authors of three major field studies concluded that diets were related to both blood cholesterol levels and CHD death rates. These conclusions were frequently referred to by the NHLBI/AHA alliance, yet the results of the studies were not at all consistent with the authors' conclusions - in fact the data should have resulted in **opposite** conclusions: (1) It was admitted that differences in diagnosing

CHD were used. (2) The total or all-cause death rates in the groups ingesting the lowest amount of saturated fat were higher than those ingesting the highest amount. (3) Cholesterol levels of several of the groups had changed substantially in follow-ups after the studies were started. Correlating original cholesterol levels with CHD death rates 10 to 15 years later was thus nonsense. (4) The relationships between blood cholesterol level and CHD were extremely weak and, because of the above, highly suspect. (5) Whereas it was maintained that one group consumed more cholesterol and saturated fat than a comparison group, the published data show the opposite to be the case.[1]

Much publicized by the alliance is the reference to the Japanese diet as being protective against disease; the Japanese are supposed to eat less fat. Drs. Robert Levy and Manning Feinleib reported that the CHD mortality rate in Japan had decreased about 20% from 1969 to 1977. They did not mention, however, that the percentage of saturated and total fat in the Japanese diet had increased.[1]

"It is painfully obvious in some instances that preconceived beliefs were to be supported no matter how much the data had to be manipulated and erroneously interpreted to achieve this end," bemoans Dr. Smith.[1]

Over 24 major studies examined individual populations in many countries over time. Even though the consumption of fats and cholesterol varied tremendously between individuals, no associations were found between individual diets and blood cholesterol levels. Dr. Basil Rifkind of the NHLBI and his colleagues admitted that "investigations within general populations seldom suggest any relation between the intake of dietary fats and blood lipid (cholesterol) concentrations."[1]

The French Paradox

The French invented Bearnaise sauce – three egg yolks and a half a pound of butter – and pour it over a fat-marbled steak. They eat flaky croissants with creamy Bries. Chickens, pork, oysters and shrimp, creamy cheeses, and other foods rich in cholesterol and saturated fat are common, everyday fare. Although the French diet would strike terror and disgust in the heart of any registered dietician in the US, France has the lowest rate of heart disease of any Western industrial-

17

ized nation. Scientific data provides copious evidence of this fact. For middle-aged men, the death rate from heart disease in France is **95** per 100,000 men; in the US it is **256** per 100,000 men. The French eat at least as much saturated fat as Americans. Their blood cholesterol levels are about the same. They outlive Americans by nearly a year.

The French have been getting 40% of their calories from fat since at least 1965 (when data began being collected). In 1974, the figure climbed to 42%. A high fat diet in that country is not new. If the cholesterol/CHD theory was correct, there has been plenty of time for atherosclerosis and heart attacks to soar!

Curtis Ellison, a Boston University epidemiologist, explains that, according to the cholesterol theory, "When you're talking about increases in fat in the diet, you don't have to wait ten to twenty years to start seeing more heart attacks and more deaths. Twenty months is more like it." So far, after at least 15 years of records, the death rate from heart disease is well below half the US rate.

Some researchers and many media reports claim that wine is the key to good heart health in the French. The alcohol itself or another chemical in wine is thought to be the key to lowering coronary risk. However, in 1990 only 23% of people over age 14 in France drank wine every day or nearly every day. Of those surveyed, 52% said they never drank wine at all.

Cheese contains more saturated fat than beef or pork. France, Italy, and Switzerland - some of the countries with the lowest heart disease rates - are among the world's leading consumers of cheese. The French top the list with each person eating about 50 pounds a year (in the US it is about 25 pounds a year). Southern France is the region with the lowest heart disease rate and it consumes the most cheese.

Regardless, over and over, researchers try to prove that if people cut their intake of cholesterol and fat, they will cut their rate of heart disease. Walter Willett, a highly respected epidemiologist at Harvard University, admits: "You'd expect that after forty years at least a handful of studies would have been conclusive, but the evidence just isn't there. Most of the studies don't show any clear effects at all." *(Nutritional Epidemiology)*

18

The World Health Organization has uncovered more puzzling facts. They considered three regions in France: (I) northern France, the land of beer and butter near Belgium, (2) eastern France, the land of pork and sauerkraut near Germany, and (3) southern France, the land of olive oil and foie gras. The cholesterol levels in the south average about midway between those of the north and east. But the rate of death from heart disease is lowest in the southern region.[38]

The attempts to link dietary cholesterol, blood cholesterol levels, and heart disease are futile because, as has been shown over and over, there is no connection.

Fat, Cholesterol and CHD

People on the island of Crete are the longest-lived people in Europe today. The heart disease rate is as low as Japan's – very small – but the people get around 40% of their calories from fat.[38] The traditional diet of the Eskimo consists largely of fish, seal, and whale blubber, yet these people do not suffer from heart disease.[35] The major foods of the Masai tribe in Tanganyika, East Africa, are meat, blood, and milk from their cattle; the fat content of their milk is twice that in the US. In spite of their high-saturated fat, high cholesterol diet, they have very low blood cholesterol levels, lower than those of surrounding tribes whose diets are more "normal." Their average blood cholesterol is 125 mg and heart disease there is virtually nonexistent. Persons over 65 who die accidentally show almost no evidence of atherosclerosis.

Some islanders in the South Pacific consume large amounts, sometimes up to 50% of their diet, of coconut oil, which is very saturated. These people have no heart or artery disease.[14] Camel herdsmen in Somali consume five quarts of camel's milk each day. Their blood cholesterol levels are no higher than 153. No heart disease is found.[11] If eating high levels of saturated fat and cholesterol are the primary dietary causes of CHD, why do all these people break the rule? Could it be that the cause of CHD has nothing to do with cholesterol?

For every report of a group of people who supposedly have a high risk of CHD because they eat high fat and high-cholesterol foods, there is another group of people who eat the same foods and have very little CHD.

19

Dr. Stewart Wolf of the University of Texas, and John Bruhn of the University of Oklahoma Medical School, analyzed more than 100 scientific articles from all over the world to find a common denominator that could be a risk factor for CHD. "They could find no consistent pattern about a certain kind of fat or a particular cholesterol level that seemed to cause heart disease."[39]

After reviewing dietary cholesterol experiments, Dr. Russell L. Smith concluded that "dietary cholesterol is unequivocally not a significant and practical factor in elevating blood cholesterol. There are only trivial theoretical health benefits and probably no real benefits to be obtained from eliminating all cholesterol from one's diet and not even theoretical benefits from eliminating 200 to 300 mg."

Fats in the Diet

All fats are made of different amounts of three fatty acids: saturated, monounsaturated, and polyunsaturated. Saturated fatty acids contain all the hydrogen atoms they can hold. Monounsaturated fatty acids are missing a pair of hydrogen atoms. Polyunsaturated fatty acids are missing two or more pairs of hydrogen atoms.

Animal fats, as in meats, eggs, milk, cheese, butter, etc., are primarily saturated and monounsaturated but do contain some polyunsaturated fatty acids. Most vegetable fats, as in vegetable oils, nuts, peanuts, etc., are primarily monounsaturated and polyunsaturated but contain some saturated fatty acids too. There are a few exceptions; for example, coconut oil, palm oil, palm kernel oil, and cocoa oil – four vegetable fats – contain mostly saturated and monounsaturated fatty acids.

All monounsaturated and polyunsaturated fatty acids are liquid at room temperature. Some saturated fatty acids are liquid at room temperature and some are solid. Monounsaturated and polyunsaturated oils become rancid over time when exposed to air (oxidized). Saturated fatty acids resist rancidity a bit more. For commercial reasons (sales and shelf life), these differences in solidity and tendency to spoil (rancidity) are very important and are the reasons for the process of hydrogenation.

Hydrogenation converts vegetable oils into solid fats by adding hydrogen atoms to the monounsaturated and polyunsaturated fatty acids, making them more saturated. A small amount of hydrogenation (partial hydrogenation) makes vegetable oils more resistant to oxidative rancidity, providing many foods (cakes, pies, crackers, breads, French fries, chips, and dozens of others) with a longer shelf life. More hydrogenation actually solidifies vegetable oils (for example, margarine and shortening) to desired consistency. Palm and coconut oils are already highly saturated, so they have been used in many baked goods with little or no need of hydrogenation.

For many years, the public has been informed of the beneficial and "curative" powers of vegetable fats. One worrisome result is the increased use of partially-hydrogenated and hydrogenated fats in the American diet. Hydrogenation converts **natural** "cis" fatty acids into **unnatural** "trans" fatty acids.

In 1990, Dutch researchers found that consuming 33 grams of trans fats each day for three weeks raised cholesterol. The US Department of Agriculture, evidently hoping to disprove the Dutch findings, carried out a study for the Institute of Shortening and Edible Oils. The people participating in the study were fed about as much **trans** fats as they get from a typical American diet. After six weeks, cholesterol levels rose higher than they did on a diet of monounsaturated fats.[40]

Trans fatty acids are harmful because they are unnatural and the body cannot process or use them as natural fats. One stress reaction to this is an increase in the blood level of cholesterol as a part of the natural effort to deal with the insult.

Intake of **trans** fatty acids has been found to increase LDL (so-called "bad") cholesterol and decrease HDL (so-called "good") cholesterol. On the basis of the current cholesterol theory, results of such studies "suggest" that the amount of **trans** fatty acids in the US diet - primarily in the form of processed vegetable fats - elevates blood cholesterol levels and increases the risk for heart attack (myocardial infarction) by at least 27%![41]

A study published in the *New England Journal of Medicine* found that hydrogenated or hardened vegetable oil, the major ingredient of margarine, "may be" worse than saturated fats in raising cholesterol, especially by raising the supposed harmful LDLs and lowering the supposed beneficial HDLs. The effects of hydrogenated vegetable fats on human health are "particularly worrisome," said the article.

"We are now faced with the paradox that a saturated fatty acid, stearic acid, does not increase serum cholesterol levels, whereas mono-unsaturated fatty acids of the trans variety do." In other words, steak, eggs, and butter are fine but margarine and other hydrogenated vegetable fats are not. "It is no longer justifiable to identify 'saturated fatty acid' as the dietary culprit responsible for raising LDL cholesterol levels."[42]

It has become a dilemma for most people to ascertain what type or types of fats to eat. The effects of many fats such as different saturated fatty acids on cholesterol are admitted to be "largely unknown" and that "too many questions are unanswered to quantitate these differences."[43] Perhaps the answer is to eat unaltered fats as nature intended including those in meats, eggs, butter, and other wholesome foods.

A recent study from Harvard Medical School linked **trans** fats to higher risk of CHD. "Intakes of foods that are major sources of **trans** isomers (margarine, cookies [biscuits], cake, and white bread) were each significantly associated with higher risks of CHD." Those who consumed the most **trans** fats had a 50% higher risk of CHD than those who consumed the least amount. The researchers' findings were admittedly a cause for increased concern regarding the use of partially-hydrogenated vegetable oils which "may have reduced the anticipated benefits of substituting these oils for highly saturated fats, and instead contributed to the occurrence of CHD."

Regardless of the overwhelming evidence, these researchers did not recommend that people switch back to butter, but rather to put olive oil on their bread or eat it plain. No matter what the facts show, the cholesterol theory must be upheld.[44]

Sugar Consumption

Another factor that might have been considered in the above Harvard Medical Study and other studies is the refined sugars (sucrose, corn syrup, fructose, sorbitol, dextrose, etc.) that appear in most foods that contain partially-hydrogenated and hydrogenated fats. One researcher showed that providing refined sugar in a water solution caused a number of species of animals on otherwise adequate diets to become so malnourished that they died.[45]

Natural, unprocessed foods contain nutrients which are important to all tissues and every physiological process in the body. Refined sugars and other highly processed foods use up nutrients; they contain very little if any nutrients themselves, and only provide calories. This depletes the body of nutrients necessary for the strength and proper elasticity of the blood vessels and for the health and contractile function of the heart muscle, as well as proper nerve transmission, for instance.

Dr. B. Friend studied food supplies in the US from 1909 to 1965. He found that, during that time, consumption of animal fats decreased while consumption of sucrose (table sugar) increased.[46] Another researcher, David Call, showed a significant reduction in milk, fat, beef fat and pork fat consumption from 1940 to 1965 and a concurrent increase in consumption of margarine, shortening, other vegetables fats and oils. During that time, CHD dramatically increased.[47]

"Animal fat consumption, which is supposed to increase CHD, decreased 20% during the time of the CHD explosion. However, during that time, sugar consumption levels increased 59%."[14]

Researcher Alfredo Lopez reviewed the work of several authors and found that, as sucrose (table sugar) consumption increased and complex carbohydrates (fruits, vegetables, whole grains, beans) decreased, the levels of both cholesterol and triglycerides in the blood rose. He then compared average blood cholesterol to consumption of sugar in people of various countries. He discovered that the relationship between dietary fat and blood cholesterol was statistically insignificant. But he did find a highly significant relationship between the level of refined sugar consumption and blood cholesterol levels. For example, Spain and Ethiopia are two countries with high fat consumption but low blood cholesterol levels. They also had very low sugar consumption. Chile and Venezuela, on the other hand, have high sugar consumption, low fat consumption, and high blood cholesterol levels. Another interesting discovery was made. When complex carbohydrate consumption was increased, there was a dramatic decrease in blood cholesterol levels.[48]

John Yudkin analyzed the refined sugar consumption of men with atherosclerosis. The men who had heart attacks ate almost twice as much sugar as those not having heart attacks. In fact, in persons with

CHD, the degree of atherosclerosis was proportional to the amount of refined sugar consumed.[49]

Coronary thrombosis in CHD is described by Dr. T.L. Cleave as one of several diseases coming into prominence during this century which is caused by the consumption of refined carbohydrate foods, especially sucrose. "Cleave received loud acclaim for his research but his teaching receives no mention today..." no doubt because it is unpopular and not in agreement with the cholesterol theory.[50]

Cuba, with one of the highest levels of sucrose consumption, has a higher death rate from heart attack (acute myocardial infarction) in men between the ages of 55 and 64 than the US. And "why are we not reminded, in pondering the fall in coronary thrombosis deaths in the USA, that sugar consumption in that country appears to have fallen from 47 kg [about 103 pounds] per person in 1958 to 32.7 kg [about 72 pounds] in 1987?"[50]

Most deaths in Caribbean countries come as a result of diabetes, hypertension, and coronary artery disease (CHD) with cancer, yet the consumption of fat is very low, about 24% of total calories. They do, however, eat a lot of refined sugars.[51]

Clinical Trials

A clinical trial is composed of two groups of similar subjects or participants. In cholesterol trials, one group receives a cholesterol-lowering treatment ("treatment" group) and the other group does not ("control" group). The subjects should be randomly assigned to the groups; if this is not done, differences between the groups later on may be as much or more due to the groups being dissimilar in the beginning rather than due to the treatment. The trial should also be "blind" in that the physicians examining the participants must not know which group they are in to avoid preconceived beliefs biasing their diagnoses.

Dr. Russell L. Smith reviewed 33 published trials. Six are rarely, if ever, mentioned by any reviewer since the articles on the trials were poorly documented, omitted important details and/or provided no evidence that the trials were randomized and blinded. The remaining 27 trials are not mentioned very often because they provide little or no support for the cholesterol/CHD relationship. Of the 27, 15 placed the treatment group on special diets to lower blood cholesterol levels; only 8 of these were both randomized and blinded and none of these showed any differences between groups in total deaths, CHD deaths or non-fatal CHD 'events' (such as heart attacks). The 7 trials left over from the 15 showed that cholesterol-lowering diets were effective, but they were not randomized, not blinded, or both. "Thus, it is hardly coincidental that when biases are permitted to influence results, the results are far different than when the biases are eliminated by design."[1] In 12 trials drugs were used to lower blood cholesterol. Only 8 were both randomized and blinded; of these, 6 had total deaths the same or **greater** in the treatment group than in the control groups; 2 of the 8 trials were considered "successful" even though total deaths were the same in both groups. Still, it is these two trials which are used for the basis of the alliance's "National Cholesterol Education Program."

Total or all-cause deaths are the bottom line of clinical trials. Of all the 27 biased and unbiased trials, 23 showed all-cause death rates the same in both treatment and control groups. Two more trials are suspect (one conducted by a pharmaceutical company to evaluate its own cholesterol-lowering drug, and the other involved an estrogen drug which produced more harm than good in three other trials). This leaves only two trials that may be considered as demonstrating a lower all-cause death rate in treatment groups. "If you had dinner in a restaurant 27 times and contracted food poisoning after 25 of these visits, would you feel confident about a 28th visit? Of course not – but then you don't think the way the NHLBI/AHA alliance thinks. No matter how many unsuccessful trials are performed, one 'successful' trial is all that the alliance needs to be correct," says Dr. Smith. And the "success" is considered to be a failure by many scientists examining the facts. Even if it were a true success, 25 unsuccessful trials cannot be overruled by one or two successful trials. Whatever happened to scientific reasoning?[1]

Of the 33 trials reviewed by Dr. Smith, two were considered by the NHLBI/AHA alliance as "conclusively" proving that lowering blood cholesterol levels reduces the rate of CHD even though all-cause deaths, CHD deaths, and non-fatal CHD events were not "significantly different" in the treatment and control groups.

The first trial was the Lipid Research Clinics Coronary Primary (LRC trial) which began in 1973 and ended in 1983; it cost $150 million. Only Caucasian men with a specific genetic disorder for high blood cholesterol levels were included – not a representation of the American population! Dietary cholesterol and saturated fat were not tested since all participants were on a low cholesterol, low saturated fat diet. Only the effect of the cholesterol-lowering drug, cholestyramine (Questran, Cholybar) was tested. The control group was given a placebo.

CHD mortality was reduced by 24%, and cholesterol blood levels were lowered about 19%. However, total mortality was virtually unchanged. Non-heart disease death rates increased by about the same amount that death rates from heart disease decreased. Those on the drug therapy experienced an increase in suicide and violent death of all types (300% higher in men treated with the drug than in the men not receiving the drug). The LRC researchers reported a 33% increase in non-cardiac mortality. Some of the frightening adverse effects of the drug included: 800% more deaths from all types of cancers including gastrointestinal cancer; 45% more incidence of gallstones, the majority requiring surgery; 100% more homicides, and 200% more accidents. All these were dismissed as "a chance occurrence" by the investigators. For obvious reasons, the so-called good results of the study were reported in the media, and the dangerous and deadly results were not mentioned.

Many researchers charged that the LRC investigators made the results look more favorable by exaggerating "statistically insignificant" data. For example, looking at actual risk, "more than seven years of treatment had reduced the chances of experiencing a heart attack from eight percent to seven percent."

It is often implied that the LRC trial proved that the reduction of cholesterol and saturated fat in the diet results in reduced mortality from CHD. How could this be since this large trial did not even test the effect of diet? The LRC trial authors stated that: "The trial's implications could and should be extended to other age groups and women, and...to others with more modest elevation of cholesterol levels." With no proof, they 'extended' their advice to almost everyone! These investigators said that the original justification for the trial was to obtain a conclusive result; although many clinical trials had been conducted to try to prove that lowering blood cholesterol level lowers CHD incidence, results had been inconclusive. After the results of the LRC trial were tabulated, though, statistical significance "could not be found using the originally agreed-upon test." So those in charge changed the test in order that statistical significance could be found. One way or another, the results were going to be what they wanted. The LRC trial did not prove a thing about cholesterol.

The second "conclusive" study was the Helsinki Trial, a virtual carbon copy of the LRC trial. This time the trial lasted 5 years; 4,081 male subjects with a specific genetic disorder were selected; blood cholesterol levels averaged 289 mg. The treatment group received the cholesterol-lowering drug, gemfibrozil (Lopid), while the control group took a placebo. The trial was funded by the pharmaceutical company that manufactures gemfibrozil.

Like the LRC authors, the Helsinki authors presented "risks" rather than rates. The actual rate difference for lowering CHD deaths was 0.26% (very insignificant). But, using "risks," the difference was amazingly converted to 26% instead - 100 times more than the absolute rate! The **actual** rate differences between the treatment and control groups for non-fatal CHD events and the combined fatal and non-fatal CHD events were only 1.2% and 1.4% respectively (also statistically insignificant). Yet the public was told that the differences were 35% and 27%!

The increase in total mortality in the Helsinki study was essentially the same. An increase in non-coronary heart disease mortality in those receiving the drug occurred from such problems as cancer, stroke (brain hemorrhage), violent death, and accidents. There was a 34% increase in non-cardiac mortality with more than double the number of deaths from accidents and violence. The total all-cause deaths (as in the LRC study) were the same in both groups in the Helsinki trial.

In sum, "the results of the two 'conclusive' trials were far from impressive. Nevertheless, the alliance classified them as highly successful." And, apparently, significant increases in accidental deaths, suicides, and cancer were not considered important.[1, 14, 52, 53, 35]

Dangers of Low Blood Cholesterol and Cholesterol-Lowering Drugs

Professor Michael F. Oliver, FRCP, of the Wynn Institute for Metabolic Research, acknowledges that many clinical trials over the last 25 years have shown reduced rates of non-fatal myocardial infarction (heart attack) but "the fall in cardiac mortality (death) is less impressive." Present data indicate that total mortality is unchanged when blood cholesterol is lowered; the "apparent" fall in CHD mortality is offset by an increase in non-cardiac deaths. "These findings can no longer be dismissed as a statistical quirk which will hopefully disappear when new trials are reported," the Professor states. "The problem was first raised in 1978 and has been observed consistently since." He also stresses that people with **naturally** low cholesterol do not have these excessive non-cardiac death rates; the problems appear when blood cholesterol is purposefully reduced. Therefore, exhorting everyone to reduce their blood cholesterol concentrations "may be premature" since the question from 25 years of experiments is whether reducing previously higher cholesterol concentrations is always safe. Professor Oliver reminds us of the maxim for physicians to "first do no harm."[53]

For six years, medical histories of 3,806 men with high blood cholesterol levels were followed. The treatment group received the cholesterol-lowering drug, cholestyramine (Questran), and the control group received a placebo. The total death rates for those on the medication was only slightly less than those on the placebo. However, those on the medication had an increase in mouth and throat cancer, colo-rectal tumors, and gallbladder disease which required surgery.[54]

Patients receiving the cholesterol-lowering drug lovastatin (Mevacor) alone or in combination with cyclosporine (Sand immune), erythromycin, gemfibrozil (Lopid), or niacin (the synthetic form of niacinamide) may develop severe rhabdomyolysis. Rhabdomyolysis is an acute, sometimes fatal disease characterized by destruction of skeletal muscle.[55]

Long-term therapy with cholesterol-lowering drugs such as colestipol (Colestid) may lower beta-carotene levels and thus increase the risk for developing some forms of cancer.[56]

Lovastatin (Mevacor) has been found to interfere with the production of ubiquinone (coenzyme Q10). Actually, lovastatin interferes with the synthesis (production) of both cholesterol and coenzyme Q10. Coenzyme Q10 is important to heart health and, ironically enough, is thought to aid vitamin E in preventing the oxidation of the so-called "bad" cholesterol, LDL, which is supposed to 'clog' arteries. People with atherosclerosis and heart disease are usually the people given cholesterol-lowering drugs like lovastatin. Thus, this must be considered adding insult to injury![57]

Lovastatin administration has also been linked to a lupus-like syndrome with "unexpected" musculoskeletal pain, stiffness, tenderness, or weakness, malaise or fever.[58]

Drugs like lovastatin and pravastatin (Pravachol) can cause a musculoskeletal reaction.[59]

Niacin, the synthetic form of a B-complex constituent, niacinamide, is used in pharmacological doses to lower blood cholesterol. Liver damage with hypothermia and metabolic acidosis has occurred with its utilization.[60]

Dr. Warren S. Browner (M.D., M.P.H.) and his associates at the University of California, San Francisco School of Medicine, applauded the Food and Drug Administration's efforts to ensure accuracy in food labeling. "Perhaps they would also improve the labeling of the cholesterol-lowering drugs currently available," they add, because, according to present data, "none of the drugs have been shown to decrease total mortality in primary prevention trials, some have actually been shown to increase noncardiovascular mortality, and one reduced high-density lipoprotein [the so-called "good"] cholesterol levels and caused substantial toxic effects in animals, while the effects of the most popular drug on disease outcomes are not known."[61]

A Finnish trial conducted by T.E. Standberg, et al, had an unexpected finding: a trivial and temporary lowering of blood cholesterol concentrations created an excess risk of CHD after the trial was completed and "doomed the subjects to long-term, increased mortality." Following participants' progress or decline after a cholesterol-lowering trial is revealing. "As we now know, 15 years are needed to document the real hazards of cholesterol reduction," commented Thomas J. Bassler, M.D. and Thomas J. Bassler, Jr., M.D. Sixty million Americans are "targeted" for cholesterol reduction at this time. The Basslers projected the results of the Finnish trial into this group and found that about 2 million of these people would die if treatment is prescribed. An analysis of many cholesterol-lowering trials "has shown a consistent increase in violent death," stated Thomas B. Newman, M.D., M.P.H., and associates, a fact that "should not be swept under the rug." These doctors believe the public should be able to reasonably expect that adhering to cholesterol-lowering recommendations would not increase their mortality, but this certainly "is no longer possible for recommendations to lower blood cholesterol levels for primary prevention of CHD." In other words, following the present recommendations or treatments to lower blood cholesterol cannot be said to prevent CHD or death - it may be hazardous to one's health and life! This is not just because of one trial such as the Finnish trial, but because of the "totality of the evidence on adverse effects of cholesterol reduction in those without known heart disease."[62]

P.B.S. Fowler of Charing Cross Hospital, London, stresses that cholesterol lowering drugs benefit the pharmaceutical industry and the academic departments that they support. It is an "unwarranted assumption" that lowering blood cholesterol levels decreases mortality, thus Dr. Fowler suggests that: "It seems a good time to halt the widespread use of various drugs and diets and consider physiological methods of reducing ischaemic heart disease [CHD]..."[63]

Cholesterol, among its other functions, is imperative to membrane tissues in the brain (synaptosomes [sacs] that break away from axon terminals at a synapse or site of functional placement between neurons). Dr. Ronan M. Conroy of the Royal College of Surgeons in Ireland provides a possible reason why increased risk of suicide and aggression occurs with lowered blood cholesterol. Since the membrane cholesterol exchanges freely with cholesterol in the surrounding internal environment, "lowered serum cholesterol may contribute to decreased brain serotonin." Serotonin is a neurotransmitter or nerve cell messenger. "Abnormalities in serotonin metabolism are associated with poor impulse control, manifest as aggression towards others or suicide." Lowering cholesterol increases violent deaths. Dr. Conroy soberly concludes that: "What is clear already is that the effects of reducing cholesterol are more subtle and far-reaching than we once thought."[64]

Albertine J. Schuit and associates, Department of Epidemiology and Public Health, Agricultural University, Netherlands, also find, via studies, that low serum cholesterol "may contribute to depletion of brain serotonin, leading to poorer suppression of aggressive behavior."[29] They have additional evidence that indicates long-term low blood cholesterol levels pose a risk for death not related to illness.[65] A 12-year study of 351,000 men (Multiple Risk Factor Intervention) reported in the *Archives of Internal Medicine* (July 1992) found that individuals with serum cholesterol concentrations under 160 sometimes develop personality changes, such as aggression, have increased risk of digestive disease, and are more likely to die from non-heart-disease causes such as cerebral hemorrhage, alcoholism, and liver and pancreatic cancer.[66]

A huge review (523,737 men and 124,814 women in the US, Japan, Europe, and Israel) was published in the American Medical Association's journal, *Circulation* (September 1990). The 13 authors of the 19 studies on cholesterol and health are uncertain as how to evaluate the findings. For example: (1) In women, cholesterol levels seem to have no influence on how often they died from all diseases. (2) In men, only those with very high or very low blood cholesterol died more often. The 64% of US men with "moderate to borderline-high" cholesterol concentrations did not die any more often or any less often. In an editorial accompanying this report, Dr. Stephen Hulley of the University of California at San Francisco, strongly recommended that cholesterol-lowering drugs not be used except in persons with evidence of heart disease already. He questioned the wisdom of even trying to lower blood cholesterol levels in women or in screening women for cholesterol levels unless they have "marked risk factors for coronary heart disease." These are amazing recommendations from someone associated with the American Medical Association![67]

In 1980, Dr. Robert Beaglehole and his colleagues reported in the *British Medical Journal* of a study involving over 600 persons in New Zealand (all with at least half native Maori ancestry). Low blood cholesterol levels (under 200 mg) paralleled greater than normal mortality due to cancer and other causes of death. In 1981, Dr. P. Oster and associates studied low blood cholesterol (less than 120 mg); the mortality in the 200 people studied was 32%. In particular, prognosis was very poor in heart disease (36%), liver disease (31%), and with malignancy (33%). They concluded "...it appears that in our population severe hypocholesterolemia [low blood cholesterol] usually is a sign of severe and possibly life-threatening disease." Dr. E. Cheraskin, M.D., D.M.D., after many years of studying cholesterol and its effects, feels one point is crystal clear: "... what evidence there is suggests that, when studied more extensively, every cell, tissue, organ and site will reflect pathology [disease] associated with hypocholesterolemia [low blood cholesterol]."[68]

Yet we are led to believe by the media that cholesterol is bad — the enemy — and the lower our blood level, the better. The truth is, from all the evidence, that this is not only false and misleading, but dangerous as well.

"Low-fat diets which successfully reduce LDL-cholesterol levels may aggravate insulin resistance associated with a greater risk of cardiovascular heart disease." For those with the tendency, lowering blood cholesterol adversely affects blood sugar (glucose) handling and increases the chance of CHD![69]

Stephen Phinney, a nutrition researcher, and his colleagues at the University of California put 44 men and women who were all 40 pounds or more overweight on very restrictive diets, low-fat and with just 400 to 600 calories a day. Blood cholesterol levels were followed. At first, their cholesterol levels fell about 10 to 20 milligrams. But four months into the diet, cholesterol levels rose by 10 to 30 milligrams on the average. One 200-pound woman began the diet with a 220 cholesterol level; she lost 70 pounds and her cholesterol increased to 422 milligrams! Once the dieters resumed a more normal diet, cholesterol levels balanced out. Ironically, Phinney's advise was still to lose weight in order to lower cholesterol.[70]

Results from a study at the University of California, San Diego, showed that low serum cholesterol may cause depression in old age. For men over 70, depression was three times as common in those with low blood cholesterol than those with normal or high cholesterol levels. The possibility of low levels of the neurotransmitter, serotonin, which are associated with depression is being considered as the reason. Animal studies already indicate that low serum cholesterol may contribute to low serotonin levels.[71]

From 1991 to 1992, 787 men and women in Nantes, France, were examined and cholesterol concentrations were studied. For both sexes, those in the group with lowest cholesterol levels had more than twice the risk of symptoms of depression than all the others. Further analyses were done in those on and off cholesterol-lowering drugs and those on and off mood-altering drugs. The results were the same – the lower the cholesterol, the better the chance for depression.[72]

An analysis of elderly men and women with malignant diseases (cancer) for three years found that cholesterol fell significantly within the year of death compared with previous years. The investigators called the association between cholesterol and malignant death "pronounced" and "sufficiently strong that it cancels out the cholesterol association with coronary death..."[73]

A group of 97 patients with "moderate hypercholesterolemia" (between 238 and 286 mg/dL) were evaluated in a recent study utilizing a low-fat diet, a high-fat diet, and low-fat diet with administration of Lovastatin (a cholesterol-lowering drug), and a high-fat diet with Lovastatin. The best results, it was expected, should have been with the low-fat/Lovastatin combination. But the results of the diet and the results of the drug were separate and independent and additive. In other words, the drug did force cholesterol levels down. "However, the reduction in LDL [so-called "bad"] cholesterol produced by the diet was small, and its benefit was possibly offset by the accompanying reduction in the level of HDL [so-called "good"] cholesterol. Merck Research Laboratories funded the study; as they are the producers of Lovastatin, the effects of the drug may have been a bit biased. Yet it was clear that the low-fat diet did not have the 'beneficial' effects desired; it didn't work.[74]

As Dr. Russell L. Smith simply states: "There is potential harm associated with the simple reduction of blood cholesterol per se and there is potential harm associated with the substances used to lower cholesterol." He cites many research studies which note possible relationships between low blood cholesterol and disease. Among the findings were: higher cancer rates and lower life expectancies. In light of this, it is dumbfounding to read such statements as that made by Dr. Carl Lavie and his colleagues in 1988 that "the risk of carcinoma [cancer] should not be used as a reason for avoiding reduction of cholesterol in the... prevention of atherosclerosis." Regardless of the fact that cholesterol has not been proven to reduce the chance of atherosclerosis, are we still to reduce cholesterol and die of cancer instead?[1]

Measuring Blood Cholesterol

In 1985 the College of American Pathologists (CAP) sent to 5,004 major hospital laboratories considered to be among the best in the US a blood sample that had a known cholesterol value of 262.6 mg. The labs, in turn, reported values ranging from 101 mg to 524 mg, a percentage difference of 318%![1]

Another study by the Center for Disease Control (CDC) showed that 52% of 130 laboratories "varied intolerably from the average."[1] Few laboratories can accurately measure HDL levels. The "finger stic" machine is also very inaccurate; even the NHLBI and the National Bureau of Standards agree. The National Bureau of Standards state "...there is currently no guarantee that a single blood test will yield an accurate picture of an individual's cholesterol level."[1]

A CAP survey in 1988 found that "about half of the nation's nearly 15,000 private laboratories **regularly** return inaccurate cholesterol measurements." (Emphasis added)

An Inspector General for the Department of Health and Human Services, Richard Kosserow, states that "an alarming number of cholesterol screenings were conducted by inadequately trained people who did not follow guidelines."[75]

A number of cholesterol tests must be performed on an individual to accurately obtain his or her average level. Different cholesterol levels will result from such things as a different physical position (sitting, standing, etc.), time of day, how the blood is drawn, and so on.

The NHLBI itself concluded that "the current state of reliability (and validity) of blood cholesterol measurements made in the U.S. suggests that considerable inaccuracy in cholesterol testing exists."[76]

Nevertheless, Americans are encouraged and frightened into having their cholesterol levels tested, and, diets and medications are prescribed on the basis of what may be an inaccurate reading of a misinterpreted test.

Inevitable Conclusions

Dr. Smith bemoans the flood of articles published in the media based on 'evidence' created by the alliance. "This literature literally seethes with contradictions, inconsistencies, illogical statements and conclusions which do not follow from the scientific data. In fact, a book could be written which is devoted exclusively to a listing of such unscientific nonsense."[1]

The sad truth is that the alliance is a "virtual economic dictatorship" within the scientific community.[1] If the research data do not support its claims, it will only create "facts" by proclaiming them to be so. Any scientist who differs with or argues against them does not receive research grants and does not get published in journals.

Additionally, much of the National Cholesterol Education Program's media blitz is financially supported by the drug and food industries – the same industries that benefit from the cholesterol scam. The American Medical Association's Executive Vice-President, Dr. James Sammons, promised physicians in 1988 of their financial rewards by stating, "the AMA's [American Medical Association's] campaign against cholesterol will bring both old and new patients to you for necessary testing, counseling and care."[1]

The *Wall Street Journal* noted that "stock ownership and other financial ties (with industries) such as consultancies, have become extensive among medical researchers."[77] Obviously a conflict of interest exists; research results would have a tendency to produce financial benefits to the drug and food industries for which the researcher has stock or other monetary interests. "If all CHD researchers were to reveal their financial ties with food and drug manufacturers, it seems unquestionable that the entire CHD research system would be viewed as completely corrupt by the public and physician practioners."[1] For example, Dr. Theodore Cooper, a former director of NHLBI, is now chairman of the board of Upjohn Pharmaceuticals, a producer of cholesterol-lowering drugs.[78]

Cholesterol screening and the development of cholesterol lowering drugs in the US alone is now a $20 billion-a-year industry.[79]

Jane Heimlich, author of *What Your Doctor Won't Tell You*, explains that she began researching the cholesterol question in 1989. She was not prepared for what she discovered – "hundreds and hundreds of medical articles protesting standard advice about cholesterol." Based on her extensive research, she is convinced that "we have been given misleading and, in some cases, harmful information about diet and drug treatment to protect the heart...[T]here is no question that the cholesterol program...benefits three powerful groups in our society to the tune of literally billions of dollars. These three are the medical profession, the pharmaceutical industry, and the food companies."[80]

Thomas J. Moore, a graduate of Cornell and a fellow of the Center for Heart Policy Research at George Washington University, is a medical journalist who exposes and debunks the so-called war on cholesterol, referring to the 30-year campaign to make the public aware of its purported dangers as a kind of medical Vietnam. It has not reduced blood cholesterol levels by much and it has not reduced coronary heart disease. The whole cholesterol uproar, according to Moore, has been tainted by ethical questions. For example, one researcher who later became a director of the National Institutes of Health bought stock in pharmaceutical company holding the patent on a cholesterol lowering drug just before announcing the results of a study favorable to the drug's effects. The editor of the AMA's publication, *Circulation*, also received stock options on the same drug company. Moore says he is also trying to expose the extent to which the medical establishment is leaning towards aggressive intervention. "The medical system is prone to going overboard. All the forces push us toward more treatment, not less. There's a new ethic that 'we gotta do something,' and it's an abrogation of the Hippocratic tradition that the physician should never do harm."[81]

Dr. Smith more adamantly declares: "The campaign to convince every American to change his or her diet and, in many cases, to initiate costly and dangerous drug 'therapy' for life is based on fabrications and monumental exaggerations of scientific findings." The NHLBI, AHA and other organizations have, as he states and proves, been involved in a conspiracy to indoctrinate the American people with a fear of cholesterol, an indoctrination costing tens of billions of dollars which will undoubtedly result in the loss of health and countless lives via cholesterol-lowering drugs, dangerously low blood cholesterol levels, and unreasonable, unhealthy diets, to say nothing of the anxiety and turmoil created.[1] Cholesterol phobia (the fear of cholesterol) is obviously a con game with monumental implications!

References

[1] Smith, Russell L., Ph.D., *The Cholesterol Conspiracy*, 1991, Warren H. Green, Inc., St. Louis.

[2] *New England Journal of Medicine*, March 28, 1991; *Science News*, Vol.139, No.15, April 13, 1991; AP release by Daniel Q. Hanley, March 28, 1991; *Health Freedom News*, January 1992; *Alternatives*, Vol.3, No.24, June 1991.

[3] *Textbook of Biochemistry with Clinical Correlations*, edited by Thomas M. Devlin, Ph.D., 1992, Wiley-Liss, NY.

[4] Bishop, Jerry E., *The Wall Street Journal*, November 18, 1992.

[5] *Science News*, Vol.143, No.5, January 30, 1993.

[6] *New England Journal of Medicine*, August 15, 1991.

[7] *Nutrition Action Healthletter*, January/February 1993.

[8] *The Lancet*, Vol.341, No.8853, May 1, 1993.

[9] *Archives of Internal Medicine*, 152 (April 1992): 775-80.

[10] Kritchevsky, David, Ph.D., "Variation in Plasma Cholesterol Levels," *Nutrition Today*, Vol.27, No.5, September/October 1992.

[11] Pinckney, Edward R., M.D., and Pinckney, Cathey, *The Cholesterol Controversy*, 1973, Sherbourne Press, Los Angeles.

[12] *Modern Medicine*, 59 (December 1991): 75; *American Journal of Cardiology*, 68.

[13] *The Lancet*, May 28, 1988, p.1237.

[14] Mudd, Chris, *Cholesterol and Your Health, The Great American Ripoff!*, 1990, American Lite Co., OK.

[15] *Internal Medicine News*, May 1 - 14, 1989.

[16] Hospitalization rates for ischemic heart disease – United States, 1970-1986, *MMWR*, 1989, 38, 275.

[17] *Acres USA*, December 1992.

[18] Douglass, William Campbell, M.D., *The Milk Book*, 1992, Second Opinion Publishing, GA, p.184.

[19] *The Lancet*, April 22, 1980.

[20] *American Journal of Clinical Nutrition*, 1970, 23:879.

[21] Taylor, William C., M.D., Beth Israel Hospital, Boston, and colleagues, *Annals of Internal Medicine*, April, 1987.

[22] Hegsted, D. Mark, Professor Emeritus of Nutrition, Harvard Schools of Medicine and Public Health, *Journal of Applied Nutrition*, 1988, 40.

[23] Kaunitz, H., Columbia University, *Journal of the American Oil Chemistry Society*, 52, August 1975.

[24] Castelli, William, M.D., *Internal Medicine News*, November 1 - 14, 1989.

[25] Livshits, Gregory, M.D., *The Journal of American Cardiology*, 1989, 63:676.

[26] *Journal of the American Medical Association*, Vol.265,No.24, June 26, 1991, p.3285-3291.

[27] *The Lancet*, Vol.337, No.8744, March 30,1991, p.787.

[28] *The American Journal of Clinical Nutrition*, Vol.50, No.1, July 1989, p.58-62.

[29] *The Lancet*, Vol.337, No.8748, April 27, 1991.

[30] Voster, Hester, H., and colleagues, *The AmericanJournal of Clinical Nutrition*, Vol.55, No.2, February 1992, p.400-410.

[31] *The American Journal of Clinical Nutrition*, Vol.56,No.5, November 1992, p.887-894.

[32] Sabete, J. et al, *New England Journal of Medicine*,March 4, 1993; Vol. 328, p.603-607.

[33] *The American Journal of Clinical Nutrition*, 53:2, 1991.

[34] *The American Journal of Clinical Nutrition*, Vol.55,No.6, June 1992, p.l060-1070.

[35] *The Doctor's People*, Vol.4, No.4, April 1991.

[36] *The Lancet*, May 11, 1985.

[37] *Nutrition Biochemistry and Metabolism*, 1st and 2nd editions, Linden, Maria C., 1985 and 1991, Elsevier, NY.

[38] Dolnick, Edward, "Beyond the French Paradox," *Health*,October 1992.

[39] Langer, Stephen, M.D. and Scheer, James F., Solved theRiddle of Illness quoted in *Health Freedom News*, July 1991.

[40] *Nutrition Action Healthletter*, Vol.19, No.10, December1992.

[41] Troisi, Rebecca et al, *The American Journal of ClinicalNutrition*, Vol.56, No.6, December 1992, p.1019-1024.

[42] *New England Journal of Medicine*, August 16, 1990.

[43] Mensink, Ronald P., *The American Journal of ClinicalNutrition*, Vol.57, No.5(S), May 1993.

[44] Willett, Walter C. et al, *The Lancet*, Vol.342, No.8845,March 6, 1993.

[45] Gigon, A.: Langdavernde Zuckerzufuhr undGlykogenbildung im Thierkorper. *Z. Ges. Exptl. Med*,. 40:1,1924.

[46] Friend, B.; *The American Journal of Clinical Nutrition*, 1967; 20:907, and updated tables, *The American Journal of Clinical Nutrition*, 1974; 27: 1.

[47] Call, David: *Trends in Fat Disappearance in the UnitedStates*, 1909 - 65; *The Journal of Nutrition*, 1967; 93(2): 1-28.

[48] Lopez, Alfredo: Some Interesting Relationships between Dietary Carbohydrates and Serum Cholesterol, *The American Journal of Clinical Nutrition*, 1966; 18: 149-53.

[49] Yudkin, John: Levels of Dietary Sucrose in Patients with Occlusive Atherosclerotic Disease, *The Lancet*, 1964; 2(7349):6-8.

[50] Cleave, T.L.: The saccharin disease. Bristol: John Wright, 1974; *The Lancet*, Vol.337, No.8748, April 27, 1991, p.1042.

[51] Hagley, K., Caribbean Food and Nutrition Institute, Kingston, Jamaica: Nutrition and Mortality Trends in the Caribbean Region: *Nutrition and Chronic Disease*; Cajanos, Vol.20, No.2, 1987.

[52] *Health Freedom News*, June 1991.

[53] *The Lancet*, Vol.337, No.8756, June 22, 1991.

[54] *Archives of Internal Medicine*, 1992; 152(7): 1399-1410.

[55] *British Medical Journal*, 1992; 304 (May 9): 1225.

[56] Mackey, S., Borchers, J., Fair, J., et al: *Circulation*, 1991; 83: 736.

[57] *Proceedings of the National Academy of Sciences*, 1990; 87: 8931.

[58] Ahmad, S., *Archives of Internal Medicine*, 1991; 151(August): 1667-1668.

[59] Schalke, B. et al, *New England Journal of Medicine*, 1992; 327 (August 27): 649-650.

[60] Dalton, T., and Berry, R., *American Journal of Medicine*, 1992; 93 (July): 102-104; *Physicians' Drug Alert*, Vol. XII, No.8, August 1991.

[61] *Journal of the American Medical Association*, Vol.267, No.3, January 15, 1992, p.363-364.

[62] Strandberg, T.E. et al, *Journal of the American Medical Association*, 1991; 266: 1225-1229. *Journal of the American Medical Association*, Vol.267, No.16, April 22/29, 1992.

[63] *The Lancet*, Vol.341, No.8840, January 30, 1993, p.314 - 315.

[64] *The Lancet*, Vol.341, No.8838, January 16, 1993, P.176.

[65] *The Lancet*, Vol.341, No.8848, March 27,1993, p.827.

[66] *Health Freedom News*, February 1993.

[67] *University of California at Berkely Wellness Letter*,Vol.9, Issue 6, March 1993.

[68] Cheraskin, E., M.D., D.M.D.: If High Blood Cholesterol is Bad - Is Low Good?, *The Journal of Orthomolecular Medicine*, Vol.1, No.3.

[69] *Nutrition Today*, January/February 1992.

[70] *In Health*, September/October 1991.

[71] *The Lancet*, Vol.341, No.8837, January 9,1993.

[72] *The Lancet*, Vol.341, No.8842, February 13, 1993, p.435.

[73] *The Lancet*, Vol.339, No.8806, June 6, 1992, p.1426.

[74] Hunninghake, D.B. et al, *New England Journal of Medicine*, Vol.328, No.17, April 29, 1993, p.1213-1219.

[75] Leary, W.E., *New York Times*, November 28, 1989.

[76] Laboratory Standardization Panel, *Clinical Chemistry*, 1988; 34, 193.

[77] Chase, M., *The Wall Street Journal*, January 26, 1989.

[78] *Health Freedom News*, April/May 1992.

[79] *World Research News*, 1st Quarter 1993, p.3.

[80] Heimlich, Jane, *What Your Doctor Won't Tell You*, 1990, Harper-Collins Publishers, NY, p. 77.

[81] Moore, Thomas J., *Lifespan*, 1993, Simon & Schuster, NY.

The Cholesterol Conundrum Continues

Between 1995 and 2010, "favorable trends" were seen in cholesterol levels. Total and low-density lipoprotein (LDL, so-called bad) cholesterol were lower, as were triglycerides. High-density lipoprotein (HDL, so-called good) cholesterol was higher. One reason is the prevalence of cholesterol-lowering drugs like statins. Prescriptions for such drugs soared during the past fifteen years—260 million prescriptions were dispensed in the United States during 2011. We're told all this is good, but the evidence begs to differ.[1]

Controversy

During the past decade, more changes (with disagreements) have been made in number "goals":

	Then (mg/dl)	Changed to	Changed again
Total cholesterol	< (less than) 240	< 200	
LDL	< (less than) 130	< 100 (2002)	< 70 (2004)
HDL	> (more than) 35	> 40	
Triglycerides	< (less than) 150	< 130	

University of Michigan scientists concluded that the new levels for cholesterol have no scientific validity but are "perhaps arbitrary." Scientific opinions **differ** on cholesterol issues or there is contrary **evidence** to theories:

- Cholesterol levels outside the "goals" increase risk for cardiovascular disease. Versus: At least **half** of all heart attacks and strokes occur in people with "desirable cholesterol levels."

- LDL/HDL **ratio** is a "valuable and standard tool" to evaluate cardiovascular risk. Versus: Individual levels of cholesterol, LDL, and HDL "are more important than the ratio."

- **New** lipid measures—lipoprotein(a) or (b), apolipoproteins, remnant-like particle cholesterol, lipoprotein-associated phospholipase A_2, etc.—may improve mathematical accuracy. Versus: It's not known which, if any, of these additional components are important, what is normal, how to use the values in practice, or whether improving the numbers reduces risk for heart disease, stroke, or anything else.

41

- **Oxidized** LDL rather than LDL per se is the problem. Versus: While oxidized LDL is found in the plaque of damaged arteries, it's less likely a cause than an **effect**. Damage to an artery lining comes before the immune response that results in plaque buildup there. Blaming LDL is like blaming a scab for the injury that caused it to form. Deficits of nutrients (vitamins A, C, and E, glutathione, etc.) that prevent premature breakdown of fats and/or consumption of altered or fake fats increase LDL oxidation.
- **Smaller**, dense LDL particles increase risk compared to larger "fluffy" ones (which "may be relatively benign"). Larger is also better for HDL particles—they're better at removing cholesterol from blood and artery walls. Versus: It's not yet known if size and density are vital. Saturated fats tend to raise levels of **large** LDL particles, "suggesting that saturated fat may not be as bad as was once thought."
- Eating fats is detrimental. Versus: Fats have not been proved to be culprits. People placed on a high-fat diet (50 percent of calories) had increases in "good" HDL but no increases in LDL beyond the levels they had on their regular diets. Actually, "blood lipid responses to the manipulation of dietary fat vary significantly between persons." Each person's response reflects his or her present needs.
- Eating cholesterol-containing **foods** increases blood cholesterol levels. Versus: Eating foods containing cholesterol usually doesn't raise cholesterol levels much or at all, but only occasionally may increase levels. A rise in cholesterol is not necessarily bad, since it indicates the body is doing work that requires cholesterol. Research hasn't shown a clear relationship between dietary cholesterol and heart disease.
- Boosting **HDL** is the most important strategy for preventing cardiovascular disease. Low HDL reduces the benefit of reducing "bad" LDL. Versus: HDL concentrations don't predict cardiovascular or any other risk. Low HDL levels "do not cause" heart attacks. People with normal HDL levels can still be at risk.
- Some people with high **HDL** and/or high **LDL** have heart

attacks; others have heart attacks with low LDL and/or low HDL. Too-low LDL is linked to anxiety, depression, cancer, and other problems. LDL is the body's early warning system, says Steve Riechman, MD, indicating something is wrong and needs to be healed. "If you did get rid of all your LDL cholesterol, you would die."[2]

Cholesterol's Functions

LDL and HDL are lipoproteins—fats combined with proteins. Since fats and watery blood don't mix well, fatty substances must be shuttled to and from tissues and cells using proteins. LDL and HDL are proteins that carry cholesterol. "There is only one cholesterol," says Ron Rosedale, MD. "There is no such thing as 'good' or 'bad' cholesterol." The liver, brain, and other cells produce cholesterol for good reasons:

- It is converted by enzymes into steroid hormones (estrogens, progesterone, testosterone, aldosterone, cortisol, etc.) Corticosteroids regulate sugar, fat, and protein metabolism.
- It is the precursor to bile acids, needed for digestion and absorption of fatty acids and fat-soluble vitamins (A, D, E, and K), without which we cannot live.
- It makes up a major part of membranes that surround cells and structures within them.
- The brain contains about 25 percent of all the cholesterol in our bodies. Myelin sheath that coats and protects nerve cells and fibers is about 20 percent cholesterol. Communication between nerve/brain cells (synapses) depends on cholesterol.
- The developing brain and eyes of the fetus and newborn infant require large amounts of cholesterol. Breast milk provides a lot of cholesterol and an enzyme to allow almost 100 percent digestion by the baby.
- Strength, energy, appetite, vitality, and gaining muscle mass depend in part on cholesterol.
- Cholesterol is needed for the immune system to properly function, preventing damage to tissues and participating in repair processes. Cholesterol is **essential** to life.

About 80 to 90 percent of cholesterol is produced in the body—the rest comes from food. When you eat more cholesterol in your diet, your body makes less. When you eat less, your body makes more. Any excess is excreted. Levels increase in winter and decrease in summer. There are fluctuations depending on time, weather, exposure to toxins, and whatever is going on in your life. Levels elevate when your body is dealing with any injury, inflammation process, or stress (physical or mental). Cholesterol increases during and after a heart attack or any other traumatic event. A woman's cholesterol levels can vary as much as 20 percent depending on what phase of her menstrual cycle she is in. Average levels are highest in women during their peri- and early menopausal years. An underactive thyroid usually results in high cholesterol levels. Obesity, insulin resistance, or diabetes will produce high cholesterol (and triglycerides). A cholesterol level too low increases risk for depression, sleep problems, aggression, violent behavior, loss of memory, poor cognition, various types of cancer, Parkinson's disease, poor immune function, increased mortality, and more.

As a repair agent, cholesterol's levels increase whenever there is insult, injury, or other need for healing. Some blood vessel areas receive more pressure and turbulence from blood flow than other areas. Plasticizers, lead, stain or water repellants, dioxins, and other toxic chemicals damage blood vessel linings or walls. Nonfoods such as refined sugars, trans fats, and others can harm blood vessels. Deficiencies of needed nutrients weaken, constrict, and stiffen blood vessels. An ongoing disease or something regularly causing damage can result in chronically high blood cholesterol levels. When any area is damaged or stressed, the liver dispatches LDL to the site to help make a "patch" and help replace damaged cells. When LDL particles are spent or finished, they're transported back to the liver by HDL where they're broken down and excreted from the body. The rationale should be to discover what is insulting, damaging, or stressing the body, requiring extra cholesterol. Forcing levels down with a drug or synthetic/isolated nutrients won't alleviate the cause—this actually interferes with repair the body is trying to accomplish. It's better to reduce the **need** for more cholesterol rather than suppress it and decrease the body's capacity to heal. Real nutritional food complexes and herbs help reduce cholesterol elevations by aiding repair, bolstering cellular function, helping to get rid of damaging agents. Then less cholesterol is needed, and levels go down. People who experience periods of acute inflammation (as in rheumatoid arthritis, lupus, or other diseases) do better if they have **higher** cholesterol levels. Those with low cholesterol levels are almost twice as likely to die of heart failure. Andrew Clark, MD, says: "In contrast to what you might imagine, having a high level of cholesterol might be good for you." Cholesterol levels may be higher when the immune system is working through any inflammation process to attempt repair. Cholesterol-lowering drugs suppress inflammation, interfering with the body's efforts to resolve damage. Ronald Kraus is a member of the committee that writes the dietary guidelines for this country. His research indicates that total cholesterol and LDL are **not** linked with heart attacks. (He did find a correlation with a specific small, dense type of LDL, but it subsided with increased consumption of saturated fat.) Most of the other members of the committee disagreed and voted to recommend the opposite. Is that science? A number of studies found **no** connection between saturated fat intake and cardiovascular disease. Although cholesterol levels are higher in North Americans than in Japanese, both populations have the same level of atherosclerosis. The cholesterol hypothesis "is like religion for some people," says Harlan Krumholz, a cardiologist at Yale University. He and others say that the cholesterol story is turning out to be messier and more nuanced than previously believed. Scientists are recognizing that HDL and LDL are not well understood. Some are asking whether HDL is even relevant to heart disease risk. Good studies are finding that lowering LDL does not prevent heart disease. People with "good" cholesterol levels have heart attacks.[3]

Statins

These cholesterol-lowering drugs (Lipitor, Mevacor, Zocor, Lescor, Crestor, Advicor, Pravachol) are being prescribed for more people than any other drug type. Some study reports sing the praises of statins for their benefits and safety. Yet virtually **all** major studies on statins were paid for or conducted by pharmaceutical companies or written by scientists with financial ties to the pharmaceutical companies producing the drugs. Statistical results are often presented in **misleading** ways, such as reporting relative risk reduction rather than absolute risk reduction. For instance, an ad boasting that Lipitor reduces heart attacks by 36 percent (relative risk) has, at the bottom in tiny print, the more accurate absolute risk: "That means in a large clinical study, 3 percent of patients taking a sugar pill or placebo had a heart attack compared to 2 percent of patients taking Lipitor." For every 100 people who took the drug for 3.3 years, 3 people on placebos and 2 people on Lipitor had heart attacks. So, 100 people have to take the drug for more than 3 years to prevent 1 heart attack. The other 99 increase their risk of side effects for nothing. Also, researchers often combine major cardiovascular events into a "composite outcome measure" that yields the most statistical power possible. This impacts the interpretation of data, but when the numbers are scrutinized, there are **no** great benefits. Data from one study show that 1,000 people would have to be treated with statins for 1 year to reduce the number of deaths from 9 to 8.

Many scientists challenge the questionable data and unfounded claims. Statins don't lower LDL in 40 percent of people taking them and "statins are not safe for all patients." Some clinical trials showed slightly lower heart disease death rates among those taking statins, but the benefit was offset by a higher rate of deaths from other causes. Any reduction in heart disease mortality is, as Uffe Ravnskov, MD, PhD, puts it, "unimpressive." Researchers ask why "the claims of benefit attributed to statin therapy in the primary prevention setting tend to be inferred from less-than-robust subset analyses or meta-analyses of clinical trials?" Real proof of benefit is lacking. Statins inhibit a liver enzyme that makes cholesterol and "poisons" everything the enzyme makes such as halting production of Coenzyme Q10 (CoQ10) and squalene. A CoQ10 deficiency can result in depression, hair loss, fatigue, cardiomyopathy, congestive heart failure, coronary artery disease, gum disease, loose teeth and more. CoQ10 supplements reduce statin-related muscle symptoms. Here are some statin **side effects**:

- Liver damage (statins inhibit production of cholesterol by the liver)
- Muscle weakness, aches, and damage; severe with higher

statin doses
- Tendonitis and tendon tears
- Increased fatigue after exertion; decline in overall energy
- Memory and cognition impairment; transient global amnesia
- Potential for depression, irritability, aggressiveness
- Damage to peripheral nerves, causing peripheral neuropathy if statins are taken longer than two years
- Lowered immune system function
- Potential increase in autoimmune diseases and cancer risk (impaired antitumor immune responses)
- Increased risk for hemorrhagic stroke
- Increase in prevalence and extent of coronary artery and aortic artery calcification
- Abdominal pain and diarrhea
- Increased risk for type two diabetes; deterioration of blood sugar control in existing diabetics
- Worsened progression and symptoms of knee osteoarthritis
- Increased risk of developing cataracts
- Sexual dysfunction
- Reduced fat metabolism including that of essential fatty acids; May suppress omega-3 benefits
- Reduction in levels of CoQ10, vitamins A, D, E, and K, and carotenes
- May deplete mineral-protein complexes including zinc, copper, selenium, and chromium
- Lactic acidosis; anemia

Most studies on statins have a high dropout rate—many people drop out because of side effects. The FDA now requires that statins carry warning labels because of the many serious adverse effects. Clinical trials of statins often find that reductions in cholesterol are not consistent with reductions in heart attacks. This led researchers to think that any ability of statins to reduce heart attacks and strokes has less to do with cholesterol reduction and more to do with plaque stability or anti-inflammatory effects. Yet lowering C-reactive protein (an inflammation marker) with statins doesn't change much. Actually, **higher** cholesterol levels protect against diseases involving lowered immune function. Edward Pickney, MD, cites twelve studies in which drugs were used to lower cholesterol; eight of the studies were both randomized and blinded. In six out of eight, deaths were greater in the treatment group than in the control group. The other four showed no differences in death rates between the control group and the treatment group. People's cholesterol levels are lower nowadays, but for men aged sixty-five to seventy-four, the rate of heart disease stayed about the same, and for people of other ages, heart disease rates have increased. Statins don't reduce risks of dying from anything.[4]

Supplements

Niacin (a synthetic form of vitamin B_3) is taken in massive doses (1,000 to 2,000 mg/day) as a drug with potential side effects (flushing, itching, nausea, blurred vision, headache, slight increases in blood sugar, liver damage, and more). Some sustained-release versions cause less flushing or less liver damage but have other adverse effects. A clinical trial in 2010 using a high-dose, extended-release niacin **and** a statin was stopped prematurely—there was a small, "unexplained" increase in ischemic strokes. Niacin raises HDL and lowers triglycerides better than statins, yet there doesn't seem to be much if any difference in reducing risks for heart attack and stroke. Niacinamide (the food form of B_3) does not cause flushing or other side effects and does not lower cholesterol like synthetic niacin—it's not a drug. **Red yeast rice** decreases total cholesterol by 13 percent and LDL by 19 percent. This fermented rice contains mevinolin, which, when isolated from the mold *Aspergillus terreus*, is a statin—lovastatin. It interferes with cholesterol synthesis and can cause the same side effects as the drug. But it doesn't appear to lower CoQ10 and may not damage muscle like statins, though elevations in liver enzymes and muscle pain do occasionally occur. Side effects include gastrointestinal discomfort, headaches, and flu-like symptoms. Red yeast rice may be safer, perhaps due to synergy with its phytochemicals. There are problems, though—it's not known how much lovastatin is in each batch, and there is possible contamination with a mycotoxin toxic to the kidneys. Red yeast rice is used as a drug with potential for harm. It shouldn't be combined with other statins due to possible additive adverse effects. **Phytosterols**, fatty substances separated from plants, are esterified and placed in foods (e.g., margarine, milk, juice, cereal, yogurt, snack bars) or capsules to lower cholesterol. Sterols occur naturally in vegetables, fruit, legumes, nuts, seeds, and grains; daily intake is 167 to 459 mg—not enough for "significant cholesterol-lowering." So sterols are given separately in huge daily doses—2,000 mg to 3,000 mg—to reduce LDL by about 9 percent. There are "strikingly" different responses to isolated phytosterols, partly depending upon the food (or nonfood) in which they are placed. They can reduce the bioavailability of carotenes and vitamins A, E, and K. When real foods with **natural** phytosterol content are eaten, cholesterol levels may eventually be reduced **if** needed because nutrients and other food factors resolve the problem for which it became elevated in the first place. High doses (600 to 900 mg) of **pantothenic acid** (vitamin B_5) lower LDL and triglycerides. B_5 can be obtained from real foods (meats, whole grains, vegetables, etc.), but doesn't have the cholesterol-lowering drug effect of the separated and synthetic version. Isolated **anthocyanin** phytochemicals, vitamin D_3 **derivatives**, and isolated soy **isoflavones** may reduce total and LDL cholesterol and slightly increase HDL—other pharmacological products. **Alpha-tocopherol, ascorbic acid**, and **beta-carotene**—all separated and synthetic chemicals—may lower cholesterol but "do not protect against cardiovascular disease." Real foods and food complexes including vitamin **E** complex, vitamin **C** complex (with rutin and flavonoids), and **carotenoids** are protective, but not as drugs. They support the strength, integrity, flexibility, and repair of blood vessel linings and walls, helping to lower the need for elevated cholesterol. **Selenium**, a component of vitamin E complex, in food such as nutritional yeast, aids in lowering cholesterol. Food **calcium** and vitamin D aid in lowering triglycerides and LDL, and in increasing HDL. **Probiotics** can reduce elevated cholesterol and LDL. **Fiber**—psyllium husks, chitosan (from crustacean shells), inulin, glucomannan, or beta glucan (from oats and barley)—may lower total and LDL cholesterol and raise HDL if needed. Stephanie Seneff, PhD, says that a deficiency of **cholesterol sulfate**—a water-soluble version synthesized in the skin and the precursor of vitamin D sulfate—may lead to defects in muscle metabolism, including the heart muscle. A 2008 study showed that "the sulfate ion attached to oxidized forms of cholesterol is highly protective against fatty streaks [in coronary arteries] and atherosclerosis."[5]

Herbs

Most products that have a fairly quick effect on cholesterol are isolated extracts from herbs used pharmacologically: Artichoke leaf extract inhibits cholesterol biosynthesis and LDL oxidation; 1,200 to 1,500 mg per day is taken. Catechins extracted from green tea and taken in large doses reduce total cholesterol and LDL cholesterol. Isolated isoflavones from red clover may affect lipid profiles. Curcumin extracted from turmeric can lower cholesterol. Berberine—an alkaloid from plants such as goldenseal and Oregon grape—reduces total cholesterol, LDL, and triglycerides while increasing HDL. Whole herbs such as garlic, ginger, cayenne, Siberian ginseng, guggul, bergamot, and fenugreek can help balance cholesterol levels in time by supporting the underlying cause. Reishi mushroom can lower blood lipids and fatty deposits in the liver. Herbs that support liver function such as dandelion, burdock, and Oregon grape root aid the metabolism of cholesterol.[6]

Fats

Studies reporting a link between a high-fat diet and heart disease or stroke looked only at total fat consumption and ignored other factors, such as how the fats/oils were processed, and consumption of refined sugars and flours. Trans fats (partially hydrogenated vegetable oils) substantially raise cholesterol and LDL, for example. Commercially fried foods and overprocessed, refined vegetable oils elicit toxic effects and impact cholesterol levels. But natural, unaltered oils and fats do not affect the lipid profile. Emphasis is shifting from reducing the quantity of fats to improving the **quality** of fats. Evidence shows **no** strong association between intake of saturated fat and risk of heart disease or stroke. One study found that a diet rich in saturated fatty acids (SFAs) led to a lower or a steady-state concentration of total and LDL cholesterol and an increase in HDL cholesterol. Similar effects were found in other trials with high or unrestricted intakes of SFAs. A meta-analysis of 21 studies with 347,000 participants found "no significant evidence for concluding that dietary saturated fat is associated with an increased risk of coronary heart disease or cardiovascular disease." Dr. Ronald Krauss shows that studies indicating benefits from replacing saturated fat with unsaturated fats don't prove that saturated fat causes cardiovascular disease. Two meta-analyses of **all** controlled clinical trials in which the only intervention was a change in dietary fats found **no** effect on coronary or total mortality. For years we heard that eggs, beef, pork, seafood, whole-fat milk products, and other cholesterol- or saturated fat–containing foods were deadly. Recent studies show that eggs, beef, pork, and other meats (except commercially processed meats containing chemical toxins), seafood, natural cheeses, and other previously forbidden foods **don't** cause problems and can be beneficial. "The theory that fat and cholesterol cause heart disease became widely accepted despite much evidence to the contrary," writes Stephen T. Sinatra, MD. "The number one dietary contributor to heart disease" is refined sugar. People should reduce or eliminate refined sugars and other refined carbohydrates. Refined sugars create effects that damage blood vessel walls, increase LDL and triglycerides, plus lower HDL. A low–refined carbohydrate diet that doesn't limit fat and includes whole grains, vegetables, fruits, fish, poultry, pasture-fed meats, nuts, and unaltered fats improves blood lipids better than a low-fat diet. **Omega-3** fatty acids, when isolated, don't seem to have much benefit. For example, in one study DHA (docosahexaenoic acid) by itself raised LDL; EPA (eiicosapentaenoic acid) alone had almost no effect on LDL. But food sources (such as cod liver oil, fatty fish) show definite benefits. Conjugated linoleic acid, alpha-linolenic acid, and gamma-linolenic acid are among other fatty acids in foods that help balance blood lipids.[7]

Food and Lifestyle

Elevated blood cholesterol is the result of the body producing more in response to a need (damage repair, cell formation, hormone production, etc.). Trans fats, refined and overprocessed oils, fried foods, refined grains, refined sugars, artificial sweeteners, industrial meats (with imbalanced fatty acids), and other items common to the Western diet can cause levels of total and LDL cholesterol to rise and HDL to sink because they stress and injure tissues. Drugs and drug-like substances lower cholesterol by interfering with the body's production, absorption, or use of cholesterol. Conversely, nutrients and other components of real foods improve or help heal the metabolic derangements and don't cause further damage or disruptions like drugs do. Then the body doesn't have to produce so much cholesterol or send so much to a needed area, resulting in lower blood levels. Consumption of healthful foods—vegetables, fruit, whole grains, nuts, seeds, legumes, unrefined oils, unaltered fats, "clean" meats and poultry and eggs and seafood—balance cholesterol levels better than eating a low-fat diet or avoiding the accused saturated fats. A variety of fats, not just one type (such as the promoted monounsaturated fats) is important for needed nutrients, fat metabolism, and balanced lipid levels. Making dietary changes may not change blood tests quickly. Time for repair, healing, and restoring balance will differ among individuals depending on the damage, stress level, hormones, immune function, and other areas needing support. Healthful foods, food-concentrate supplements, regular physical activity, a low toxic load (including not smoking), and manageable stress make a healthful formula to support balanced cholesterol levels and avoid heart disease and stroke.[8]

"The Cholesterol Conundrum Continues" was originally published in *Nutrition News and Views*, May/June 2013, 17(3).

[1] MD Carroll, BK Kit, et al., *JAMA*, 17 Oct 2012, 308(15):1545–54; M Mitka, *JAMA*, 22/29 Aug 2012, 308(8):750–1.
[2] *UC Berkeley Wellness Lttr*, Sept 2012, 28(13):1–2; M Gillman, S Daniels, B Psatu, et al., *JAMA*, 18 Jan 2012, 307(3):257–60; M Fernandez, D Webb, *J Am Coll Nutr*, Feb 2008, 27(1):1–5; P Gomez, P Perez-Martinez, et al., *J Nutr*, Apr 2010, 140(4):773–8; Lp-PLA Studies Collab, *Lancet*, 1 May 2010, 375(9725):1536–44; Emerging Risk Factors Collab, *JAMA*, 22/29 July 2009, 302(4):412–23 & 20 Jun 2012, 307(23):2499–2506; JY Kim, YJ Hyun, *Am J Clin Nutr*, Sept 2008, 88(3):630–7; R Bradley, E Oberg, *Integrat Med*, Jun/Jul 2011, 10(3):56–61; T Gaziano, C Young, et al., *Lancet*, 15 Mar 2008, 371 (9616):923–31; S Mendis, V Mohan, *Lancet*, 15 Mar 2008, 371(9616):878–9; *Duke Med Hlth News*, Aug 2012,

18(8):1–2; J Despres, *Lancet*, 4 Apr 2009, 373(9670):1147–8; M Mitka, *JAMA*, 4 Jan 2012, 307(1):21–2; Presentation, Am Coll of Cardiology, 61st Annual Scientific Session, Chicago, IL, 24–27 Mar 2012; A Onat, *Lancet*, 8 Dec 2012, 380(9858):1989–90; T Saey, *Sci News*, 16 Jun 2012, 181(12):14; *Tufts Univ Hlth & Nutr Lttr*, Aug 2012, 30(6):7; TX A&M Univ, http://tamunews.tamu.edu/201 1/05/04/%e2%80%98bad%e2%80%99-cholesrerol; CP Cannon, *JAMA* 16 Nov 2011, 306(19):2153–5; R Karas, et al., *J Am Coll Cardiology*, 22 Jun 2010, content. onlinejacc.org/cgicontent/abstract/55/25/2846; E Pennisi, *Science*, 25 May 2012, 336(6084):977.

3 S Mumford, et al., *J Clin Endocrinol Metab*, Sept 2010, doi: 10.1210/jc 2010-0109, 95:E80-5; J Couzin-Frankel, *Science*, 10 Jun 2011, 332(6035):1252–3; S Riechman, et al., *J Gerontology* cited in GreenMedInfo.com/cholesterol, 17 Sept 2012; A Brownawell, M Falk, *Nutr Rev*, Jun 2010, 68(6):355–64; PDS, *Science*, 20 Nov 2009, 326(5956):1043; L Lumey, A Stein, et al., *Am J Clin Nutr*, Jun 2009, 89(6):1737–43; J Couzin, *Science*, 10 Oct 2008, 322(5899):220–3;P Amarenco, P Steg, *Lancet*, 1 Dec 2007, 370(9602):1803–4; L Woollett, *Am J Clin Nutr*, Dec 2005, 82(6):1155–61; I Ockene, et al., *Arch Intern Med*, 2004, 164:863–70; 10th Report on Carcinogens, www.ehp.niehs,nih.gov; J Travis, *Sci News*, 17 Nov 2001, 160(20):309; B McDonald, *J Am Coll Nutr*, Dec 2004, 23(6):616S–20S; A Singh-Manoux, D Gimeno, et al., *Arterioscler Thromb Vasc Biol*, Aug 2008, 28(8):1556–62; X Huang, P Auinger, et al., *PLoS One*, 2011, 6(8):e22854; MD Weeks, 4 Mar 2012; Honolulu-Asia Aging Study, *Arch Neurol*, 2007, 64:103–6; J Kaplan, M Muldoon, et al., *Psychosom Med*, 2005, 67:24–30; I Schatz, et al., *Lancet*, 4 Aug 2001, 358(9279):351–5; N Schupf, R Costa, et al., *J Am Geriatr Soc*, 2005, 53.219–26.

4 M Kawashiri, A Nohara, et al., *Clin Pharmacol Ther*, 2008, 83(5):731–9; T Suzuki, T Nozawa, et al., *Int Heart J*, 2008, 49(4):423–33; L Mascitelli, F Pezzetta, *Lancet*, 31 Mar 2007, 369(9567):1078–9; A Ali-Alsheikh, P Maddukuri, et al., *J Am Coll Cardiol*, 2007, 50:409–18; P Coogan, L Rosenberg, et al., *Epidemiology*, 2007, 18:213–9; J Swartzberg, *UC Berkeley Wellness Lttr*, Nov 2012, 29(2):8; M Mohaupt, et al., *CMAG*, 7 Jul 2009; M Mitka, *JAMA*, 7 Mar 2012, 307(9):893–4; B Staels, *Lancet*, 29 May 2010, 375(9729):1847–8; D Preiss, S Seshasai, et al., *JAMA*, 22/29 Jun 2011, 305(24):2556–64; C Heneghan, *Cochrane Database Syst Rev*, 14 Jan 2011, 8:ED000017; Heart Protect Study Collab Grp, *Lancet*, 5 Feb 2011, 377(9764):469–76; M Napoli, http://medicalconsumers.org/2010/1007/statins-dont-work/; A Callahan, P Amarenco, et al., *Arch Neurology*, 2011, 68(10):1245–51; *J Infectious Dis*, Jan 2012, 205(1):13–9; A Culver, I Ockene, et al., *Arch Intern Med*, 2012, 172(2):144–52; R Redberg, M Katz, *JAMA*, 11 Apr 2012, 307(14):1491–2; M DeLorgeril, P Salen, et al., *Arch Intern Med*, 28 Jun 2010, 170(12):1032–6; G MacDonald, *JAOA*, Aug 2010, 110(8):424–5; P Redker, E Danielson, et al., *N Engl J Med*, 2008, 359(21):2195–2207; A Limprasertkul, N Fisher, et al., *J Am Coll Nutr*, Feb 2012, 31(1):32–8; B Golomb, *Sci News*, 30 Jun 2012, 181(13):31; J Rubinstein, F Aloka, et al., *Cardiol*, Dec 2009, 32(12):684–9; W Subczynski, M Ragus, et al., *J Membr Biol*, Jan 2012, 245(1):51–68; A Saremi, G Bahn, et al., *Diabetes Care*, 8 Aug 2012, Epub ahead of print; K Ray, S Seshasai,

et al., *Arch Intern Med*, 2010, 170:1024–31; P Otruba, P Kanovsky, et al., *Neuro Endocrinol Lett*, 3 Sep 2011, 32(5):688–90; S Clockaerts, G Van Osch, et al., *Ann Rheum Dis*, May 2012, 71(5):642–7; D Newman, V Saini, et al., *Lancet*, 24 Nov 2012, 380(9856):1814; N Seppa, *Sci News*, 15 Dec 2012, 182(12):9; H Ong, A Haniffah, *Lancet*, 5 Apr 2008, 371(9619):1161; M de Lorgeril, P Salen, et al., *BMC Med*, 4 Jan 2013, Epub ahead of print; S Eussen, J Geleijnse, et al., *Eur Heart J*, Jul 2012, 33(13):1582–8.

5 H Karpman, *Altern Med Alert*, Apr 2012, 15(4):47–8; J Scholle, W Baker, et al., *J Am Coll Nutr*, Oct 2009, 28(5):517–24; M Kurokawa, Y Masuda, et al., *J Oleo Sci*, 2008, 57(1):35–45; M Napoli, http://medicalconsumers.org/2011/12/11/niacin; N Plana, L Masana, et al., *Eur J Nutr* 2008, 47(1):32–9; R Acuff, D Cai, et al., *Lipids Hlth Dis*, 2007, 6:11; S Goncalves, A Maria, et al., *Nutr Res*, 2007, 27(4):2000–5; I Demonty, R Ras, et al., *J Nutr*, 2009, 139(2):271–84; X Lin, R Ostlund Jr, et al., *Am J Physiol Gastrointest Liver Physiol*, 2009, 296(4):G931–5; S AbuMweis, C Vanstone, et al., *Eur J Clin Nutr*, 2009, 63(6):747–55; I Demonty, RT Ras, et al., *J Nutr*, Feb 2009, 139(2):271–84; S Racette, X Lin, et al., *Am J Clin Nutr*, Jan 2010, 91(1):32–8; S Klingberg, L Ellegard, et al., *Am J Clin Nutr*, Apr 2008, 87(4):993–1001; C Venero, P Thompson, et al., *Am J Cardiol*, 2010, 105(5):664–6; D Becker, R Gordon, et al., *Ann Intern Med*, 2009, 150(12):830–9; S Halbert, D Becker, et al., *Am J Cardiol*, 2010, 105(2):198–204; J Li, et al., *J Clin Pharmacol*, 2009, 49:947–56; T Low Dog, *Altern & Complem Ther*, Oct 2010, 16(5):256–7; R Gordon, T Cooperman, et al., *Arch Intern Med*, 25 Oct 2010, 170(19): 1722–7; M Rayman, et al., *Ann Intern Med*, 2011, 154:656–65; ConsumerLab.com, Red yeast rice supplements, 20 May 2011; F Francini-Pesenti, et al., *Phytother Res*, 2008, 22:318–22; J Rumberger, J Napolitano, et al., *Nutr Res*, Aug 2011, 31(8):608–15; Y Qin, M Xia, et al., *Am J Clin Nutr*, Sep 2009, 90(3):485–92; R Kazlauskaite, J Calvin, et al., *J Clin Lipidol*, 2010, 4(2):113–9; R Jorde, Y Figenschau, et al., *Eur J Clin Nutr*, Dec 2010, 64(12):1457–64; K Taku, K Umegaki, et al., *Am J Clin Nutr*, Apr 2007, 85(4):1148–56; Z Guo, W Chen, et al., *Nutr Metab Cardiovasc Dis*, 17 Sep 2011, Epub ahead of print; M Fuentes, T Lajo, et al., *Br J Nutr*, 28 Sep 2012:1–7; N Sood, W Baker, et al., *Am J Clin Nutr*, Oct 2008, 88(4):1167–75; N Tapola, M Lyyra, et al., *J Am Coll Nutr*, Feb 2008, 27(1):22–30.

6 V Mollace, et al., *Fitoterapia*, Apr 2011, 82(3):309–16; A Kim, A Chiu, et al., *J Am Diet Assoc*, Nov 2011, 111(11):1720–9; M Terzic, B Tosic-Race, et al., *J Obstet Gynaecol Res*, 2009, 35(6):1091–5; Y Lee, H Kwak, et al., *Biochem Biophys Res Commun*, 28 Jul 2008; Epub ahead of print; R Bundy, H Simpson, et al., *Phytomed*, Sep 2008, 15(9):668–75; D Peschel, R Koerting, et al., *J Nutr Biochem*, 2007, 18(2):113–9; W Kong, et al., *Nat Med* 2004, 10:1344–51; A Cicero, L Rovati, et al., *Arzneimittelforschung*, 2007, 57(1):26–30; P Nestel, M Cehun, et al., *Eur J Clin Nutr*, 2004, 58:403–8; J Coon, E Ernst, *J Fam Pract*, Jun 2003, 52(6):468–78; S Coimbra, A Silva, et al., *Nutr Res*, 2006, 26(11):604–7; D Maron et al., *Arch Intern Med* 2003, 163:1448–53.

7 V Buonacorso, ER Nakandakare, et al., *Am J Clin Nutr*, Nov 2007, 86(5):1270–7; D Kim, *JAMA*, 21 Nov 2007, 298(19):2263–4; *Nutrition Week*, 16 May 2005,

5(10):4; D Katz, M Evans, et al., *Int J Cardiol*, 2005, 99:65–70; C Greene, T Zern, et al., *J Nutr*, Dec 2005, 135(12):2793–8; *UC Berkeley Wellness Lttr*, Apr 2007, 23(7):7–8; K Mayurasakorn, et al., *J Med Assoc Thai*, 2008, 91(3):400–7; A Lichtenstein, *Tufts Univ Hlth & Nutr Lttr*, Mar 2009, 27(1):7; J Hjerpsted, E leedo, et al., *Am J Clin Nutr*, Dec 2011, Epub ahead of print; *Duke Med Hlth News*, May 2012, 18(5):8; S Sinatra, *J Am Coll Nutr*, Jun 2012, 31(3):223; A Slyper, J Jurva, et al., *Am J Clin Nutr*, 2005, 81:376–9; J Welsh, A Sharma, et al., *JAMA*, 21 Apr 2010, 303(15):1490–7; Weill Cornell Med Coll, *Food & Fitness Adv*, Oct 2008, 14(10):5; R Krauss, http://keithconnectsthedots.com/2009/01/31/ronald-krauss-part2.aspx; A Merchant, S Anand, et al., *Am J Clin Nutr*, Jan 2007, 85(1):225–30; R Wood, M Fernandez, et al., *Metabolism*, 2007, 56(1):58–67; M Nikfardjam, *Lancet*, 8 Dec 2012, 380(9858):1976–7; B Raghu, P Venkatesan, *Indian J Clin Biochem*, Jan 2008, 23(1):85–8; M Wei, T Jacobson, *Curr Atheroscler Rep*, 6 Oct 2011, Epub ahead of print; S Egert, F Kannenberg, et al., *J Nutr*, May 2009, 139(5):861–8; A S-Vila, E Ros, et al., *Am J Clin Nutr*, 12 May 2010, Epub ahead of print.

8 S Rajaram, J Sabate, et al., *Am J Clin Nutr*, 2009, 89(5):1657S–63S; N Damasceno, A Perez-Heras, et al., *Nutr Metab Cardiovasc Dis*, Jun 2011, 21(S 1):14–20; R Othman, M Moghadasian, et al., *Nutr Rev*, Jun 2011, 69(6):299–309; A Bouchard-Mercier, A Paradis, et al., *J Am Coll Nutr*, Dec 2010, 29(6):630–7; B Freeman, A Linares, et al., *J Am Coll Nutr*, Feb 2010, 29(1):46–54; B Alipoor, M Haghighian, et al., *Int J Food Sci Nutr*, 23 Jan 2012, Epub ahead of print; K Torre-Carbot, J Chavez-Servin, *J Nutr*, Mar 2010, 140(3):501–8; D Jenkins, J Wong, et al., *Arch Intern Med*, 2009, 169:1046–54; A Pan, D Yu, et al., *Am J Clin Nutr*, Aug 2009, 90 (2):288097; *PLoS One*, 2012, 7:e38901; I Hatoum, J Nelson, et al., *Am J Clin Nutr*, Mar 2010, 91(3):786–93.

Cholesterol, Fats, and Heart Attacks, Part 1

At first, all cholesterol was bad; it clogged arteries and caused heart attacks. Then researchers sorted out "good" HDL cholesterol from "bad" LDL cholesterol; an unfavorable ratio increased heart attack risk. Later, particles of lipoprotein(a) and/or apolipoprotein B were implicated, followed by triglycerides. Americans were told to avoid dietary cholesterol. Then it was saturated fats. Finally, fats in general had to be reduced. What is the cholesterol/fat/heart attack connection?

Cholesterol

"Cholesterol" is not a dirty word. Cholesterol is an alcohol (though it does not behave as one) and not really a fat. It is primarily produced by the liver (though all cells are able to produce it) and travels through the bloodstream to every cell, tissue, and organ. It is needed for fat metabolism, the development of cells, as an important constituent of cell walls, to maintain the strength of blood vessel walls, to synthesize bile components, in vitamin D production, for brain function, and as a component of myelin sheath that protects nerves and nerve-impulse propagation. It is essential for strength and resilience. It is used in seminal fluid and vaginal lubrication. It is the basic substance from which steroid hormones like DHEA, cortisol, estrogen, progesterone, and testosterone are produced. It is required for normal development of embryos. Cholesterol is used to repair and protect tissues, and much more. The body goes to an awful lot of trouble to produce and balance cholesterol. It is essential for human life.

Most of the cholesterol the body needs—about 2,000 milligrams (mg) per day—is synthesized by the liver. The average American ingests between 300 to 500 mg of cholesterol per day from animal foods such as meats, eggs, seafood, and dairy products. This means 80 to 85 percent of cholesterol is produced by the liver, and only 15 to 20 percent is obtained from dietary sources. Even without the intake of cholesterol-containing foods, the body sufficiently balances cholesterol. Consumption of cholesterol-containing foods does not in and of itself cause chronically high cholesterol levels in the blood.

The amount of cholesterol produced by the liver is dependent on the total available cholesterol—regardless of the source. A feedback system reduces its production if there is more than needed. Thus, dietary cholesterol may serve to reduce its synthesis in the body. Any excess cholesterol is simply excreted through the bile. So, if one eats too much cholesterol, the cells produce less. If one eats too little, the cells produce more. It is not easy to change one's cholesterol level by changing the diet. It can be done, but only by 5 to 10 percent. About 5 percent of the population has very high blood levels of cholesterol (350 and above) probably due to a genetic metabolic disorder that "is merely reflected in high cholesterol readings—like a fever indicates an infection and is not a disease itself."[1]

Cholesterol Numbers

Blood cholesterol numbers currently used include:

Total cholesterol
> no risk: less than 150; low risk: 150 to 200; medium risk: 200 to 250; high risk: greater than 250

Low-density lipoprotein (LDL)
> no risk: less than 100; low risk: 100 to 130; medium risk: 130 to 160; high risk: greater than 160

High-density lipoprotein (HDL)
> no risk: greater than 75; low risk: 60 to 75; medium risk: 40 to 60; high risk: less than 40

Ratio of Total cholesterol/HDL
> no risk: less than 3.5; low risk 3.5 to 4.5; medium risk: 4.5 to 5.5; high risk: greater than 5.5

Another marker appearing is **triglyceride/HDL** ratio—"should be" below 2.0

Cholesterol researcher Uffe Ravnskov, MD, PhD, challenges the limit of 200 arbitrarily placed on total cholesterol back in the 1980s. "This is a level invented without any evidence." What determines the blood cholesterol level is "difficult to tell because there are so many factors that influence" it, from mental stress or anger to exercise, from weight gain or loss to tissue insults and injury. To set a limit of 200 and to proclaim that any number below that is healthy and any number above that is unhealthy is "pure speculation." It is based on the idea that cholesterol levels above 200 predict coronary heart disease. Some studies seem to show this, but others do not.

In his book, *The Cholesterol Myths*, Dr. Ravnskov provides a thorough account of numerous cholesterol studies. He reveals that some studies that seem to show a relationship between "high" cholesterol levels and coronary heart disease (CHD) include data that are inconsistent and highly questionable. In some cases, conclusions reached by researchers are completely contrary to what the data show. Research papers and reviews by organizations like the National Heart, Lung and Blood Institute and the American Heart Association "systematically ignore all contradictory evidence. They all cite the contradictory papers as if they were supportive." In some cases when researchers get results that are contrary to the cholesterol hypotheses, they write conclusions indicating that their findings support the idea. Most people (including doctors and other researchers) read only these conclusions as written in the summary. To find the contradictions, one would have to read the whole papers and meticulously study the graphs. Correlations between CHD and cholesterol levels are often weak. False correlations are not unusual. For example, a false correlation between atherosclerosis and blood cholesterol may be made when the actual relationship is between atherosclerosis and age or between cholesterol and age. Or a correlation between cholesterol and the degree of atherosclerosis may appear in studies that include people with familial hypercholesterolemia (genetically induced high cholesterol); if these participants are excluded from the statistics, the correlation disappears. Many studies have found no association between cholesterol levels and heart mortality. Some studies indicate **low** cholesterol predicts CHD.

From the rhetoric, it is assumed that people who have heart attacks almost always have large amounts of cholesterol in their blood. Yet data demonstrate that the difference between those who have CHD and those who do not is marginal. For example, a graph from the famous Framingham heart study shows that almost half of those who had a heart attack had low cholesterol. As time passed in this thirty-year study, a "few" more people with high cholesterol levels died—on average 1 percent of all men with high cholesterol died each year. Only half as many died among those with the lowest cholesterol values. Women with low cholesterol died just as often as women with high cholesterol. It appeared that high cholesterol was more dangerous, but the figures released included death from ALL causes, not just heart mortality. And, cholesterol levels made no difference for men over the age of forty-seven—those who had low cholesterol at age forty-eight and older died just as often as those with high cholesterol. Evidently, if you reach age forty-seven, it does not matter whether your cholesterol is high or low! More than 95 percent of all heart attacks occur in people older than forty-eight. If cholesterol levels are important for the few who have heart attacks before age forty-eight, why should everyone else worry about blood cholesterol levels? Actually, during the thirty-year Framingham study, those whose cholesterol had **decreased** "by itself" actually ran a greater risk of dying than those whose cholesterol had **increased**. The report stated: "For each 1 mg/dl drop of cholesterol there was an 11 percent increase in coronary and total mortality."

For many years the public has been told how important it is to lower their cholesterol levels to prevent coronary heart disease. Yet the large Framingham study demonstrated that if blood cholesterol decreases by itself, the risk of dying increases. The report clearly shows that mortality **increased**, yet the written review stated that mortality **decreased**. This was only one of many "mistakes" presented to the public.

High cholesterol in women is not a risk factor. Studies show that it is more dangerous for women to have low cholesterol than high. "Excess dietary cholesterol" does not increase the risk of developing CHD in women. Elderly women with very high cholesterol live the longest. Although high cholesterol levels appear to have a "slight association" with increased risk for men in the United States, it has no such association for men in Canada. Neither is blood cholesterol important for those who have already had a heart attack. In Russia, **low** cholesterol is associated with increased risk of CHD. In Stockholm, men with low cholesterol died from heart disease just as often as those with high cholesterol. The people of the Maasai tribe in Kenya eat a diet of milk and meat with twice the fat and cholesterol content of most Western diets, and yet they are basically free of heart disease. The Maori, Polynesians who migrated to New Zealand hundreds of years ago, may die from heart attacks, but they do so whether their cholesterol is low or high. The Batemi people of Tanzania average up to 2,000 milligrams of cholesterol a day in their diets, well over the "maximum recommended daily intake of 300 milligrams." Yet their blood cholesterol levels are low (about one-third the levels of the average American) and they do not suffer with CHD. The Mennonites, an agrarian community similar to the Amish, follow a traditional diet high in cholesterol and saturated fat—with abundant dairy products, eggs, and red meat—but have serum cholesterol and blood pressure levels lower than other Americans.

Research shows that "there is little relationship between serum cholesterol values and coronary heart disease in those over 70." **Low** blood cholesterol levels are associated with malnutrition, disease, and death, especially among the elderly. Cholesterol levels higher than "normal" are associated with increased longevity in people over age 85. With increasing age, persistence of **low** cholesterol levels increases risk of death.

Thus, high cholesterol is said to be dangerous but not for Canadians, Russians, Stockholmers, Maasais, Maoris, Batemi, or Mennonites. High cholesterol is said to be dangerous to men but not to women; dangerous for healthy men but not for those who had heart attacks; dangerous for men under age forty-seven but not those forty-eight and older. High cholesterol may even be beneficial for older people. Obviously, any association between high cholesterol and CHD is not one of simple cause and effect. "The most likely interpretation is that high cholesterol is not dangerous in itself but a marker for something else." High or low cholesterol concentrations are "not pathogenic by themselves but are secondary to other, more important factors." It follows that lowering cholesterol levels by diet does not lower the risk of heart mortality. One indication that high cholesterol is not pathogenic by itself is the percentage of people who have familial high cholesterol levels and reach a normal life span with a lower risk of CHD than the general population. There are "environmental factors of much greater importance than the cholesterol concentration."

Smoking; overweight; high blood pressure; stress; altered or damaged dietary fats; refined sugars; nutritional deficiencies; fragility, loss of elasticity, and lesions of the coronary arteries—all these have a much stronger association with CHD than cholesterol levels. Serum total cholesterol levels are elevated in liver imbalances, disease, or toxic overload; hypothyroidism; diabetes; kidney disease; and other chronic problems or stresses. "Cholesterol is nature's healing substance. Without it wounds would not heal and our cells could not maintain their integrity." Just as plant cells depend on their structure and firmness from cellulose, human cells—including cells forming blood vessels—obtain their shape and strength from cholesterol. Thus elevated cholesterol levels indicate an increased need to support, protect, or replenish when there has been insult, injury, or depletion. When lifestyle improvements including a healthier diet result in a lowering of serum cholesterol, it means that the body no longer requires the extra circulating cholesterol. The repair or protection has been completed, or the excessive stress has been reduced. For example, physical or emotional distress may induce the adrenal glands to produce larger than usual amounts of steroid hormones to cope. Increased amounts of cholesterol are needed as raw material for the hormone production. Once the distress is reduced and the adrenal glands recuperate, the need for extra cholesterol diminishes.

Back in 1990, a study from Georgetown University showed that total cholesterol levels varied by more than 20 percent in 75 percent of participants. Similarly, LDL and HDL cholesterol fluctuations of the same magnitude were found in 65 to 95 percent of the subjects. With retesting, 40 percent of the participants moved from one risk category to another, and 10 percent moved from the lowest risk category to the highest risk category or vise versa. "Fluctuations occurred randomly from week to week, and were unrelated to age, sex, or the serum levels of lipoproteins." Cholesterol numbers vary among individuals (biochemical individuality) and will change when the need for cholesterol changes. Results of a cholesterol blood test can be influenced by changes in diet, fluctuations in weight, amount of alcohol intake, injury, surgery, infection, physical strain, most any stress, and numerous other circumstances. Not only an individual's past readings must be considered to determine what is basically "normal" for him or her, but also present and varying circumstances must be taken into account. From 50 to 60 percent of all heart attacks occur in people with "acceptable" or "desirable" cholesterol levels.

Scientists admit that "not all epidemiological studies show a correlation between dietary cholesterol alone and either serum cholesterol or coronary heart disease." The "large difference in absolute CHD mortality rates at a given cholesterol level...indicates that other factors, such as diet, that are typical for cultures with a low CHD risk are also important with respect to primary prevention." In other words, serum cholesterol levels are generally meaningless when it comes to heart disease. And a healthful diet, whether or not it contains cholesterol-rich foods, is essential to prevent CHD. People with CHD and "normal" levels of cholesterol who are given cholesterol-lowering drugs respond with significantly lower serum cholesterol levels but **no "measurable benefit on the coronary arteries."** If there is no benefit to the blood vessels that are supposedly "clogged" with cholesterol, then something other than cholesterol must be causing the problem!

Indeed, the "consistency of the clinical and the epidemiological data demonstrating that dietary cholesterol has little effect on plasma cholesterol in most individuals raises a number of questions regarding the justification of population-wide restrictions on dietary cholesterol intake." Scientists, despite a vast array of cholesterol studies, have been unable "to detect associations between diet and serum cholesterol." Every cell in every animal, including humans, contains cholesterol. Animal fat, composed of animal cells, contains cholesterol. Lean meat, also composed of animal cells, contains cholesterol. Some animal foods contain more cholesterol than others. Fat does not determine the cholesterol content. For example, butter and lard are high in fat but low in cholesterol. Eggs and liver are low in fat but high in cholesterol. Eggs are now approved by heart associations and dieticians as part of a healthy, CHD-preventive diet. Natural, unaltered foods, even those high in cholesterol, do not increase risk for CHD. A low-cholesterol diet will not prevent heart attacks. The blood level of cholesterol will not determine if an individual is more likely to have a heart attack or not.[2]

Lipoproteins

What about "good" high-density lipoprotein (HDL) cholesterol and "bad" low-density lipoprotein (LDL) cholesterol?

The cholesterol molecule is arranged in an intricate network that is impossible to dissolve in water. Because it is insoluble, it circulates in the blood inside round particles made of fats (lipids) and proteins—lipoproteins. The outside of lipoproteins is composed mostly of water-soluble proteins. The inside is composed of lipids with room to carry water-insoluble molecules like cholesterol. Lipoproteins serve as "vehicles" to transport cholesterol through the blood and are categorized by their protein density (high density, low density, etc.).

The primary job of HDL is to pick up used or unneeded cholesterol molecules and cholesterol esters **from** all peripheral tissues, including artery walls, and transport or return them **to** the liver as part of a recycling process. In the liver, cholesterol is excreted with the bile or used for other purposes. When cholesterol needs to be removed from cells, it is HDL that usually does the job. Some cholesterol is always sloughing off cellular membranes into the plasma. HDL is believed to be protective, preventing a buildup of cholesterol and lowering risk of CHD by removing unused cholesterol from the blood. It is also thought that HDL may be able to collect cholesterol from artery plaque, reversing the atherosclerotic process leading to heart attacks.

The LDL particles primarily carry cholesterol **from** the liver (where most of the body's cholesterol is synthesized) **to** the peripheral tissues, including blood vessel walls. When cells need extra cholesterol, it is the LDL vehicles that deliver cholesterol into the cellular interiors. In most (not all) people, LDL contains a higher percentage of cholesterol, so has been dubbed "bad." When a cell needs more cholesterol, it produces more LDL receptors on its plasma membrane. This allows the cell to bind more LDL, ingest it, and obtain its cholesterol—a process the cell prefers over making cholesterol itself. Generally, when cells need cholesterol, LDLs come to the rescue.

Between 60 and 80 percent of cholesterol in the blood is transported by LDL. About 15 to 20 percent is carried by HDL. Smaller amounts of cholesterol are carried in circulation by other types of lipoproteins such as VLDL (very low density lipoprotein). The liver is "the center of the cholesterol universe." It synthesizes new cholesterol, recycles used cholesterol, and secretes old cholesterol into bile, transforming it into bile acids. The production of cholesterol by the liver is inhibited whenever dietary cholesterol is increased and stimulated when dietary cholesterol is reduced. This homeostatic control is the primary reason why it is actually difficult to alter plasma cholesterol very much in either direction by altering the diet. So attention was focused on the "messengers" HDL and LDL regarding CHD risk. Some health professionals point to LDL levels that are too high and HDL levels that are too low. Others consider ratios as most telling—ratios between HDL and LDL or between HDL and total cholesterol. The average U.S. ratio of total cholesterol to HDL is 5 to 1 (HDL representing one-fifth or 20 percent of total cholesterol) and is not considered healthy. A better ratio is thought to be 3 to 1—33 percent of total cholesterol. Still, many experts feel that individual levels of total cholesterol, HDL, and LDL are more important than ratios. What does it all mean?

Excess weight gain results in an increased risk of CHD as well as higher LDL and lower HDL. Lack of physical exercise, hypertension, and smoking do the same. The question is: Do these or other known CHD risk factors bring about heart attacks BECAUSE of the increased LDL and decreased HDL? Or are the changes in LDL and HDL a RESULT of insult, injury, or imbalance that triggers an increased need for cholesterol in the cells involved? When a person becomes overweight, for example, there is more stress on the heart, blood vessels, liver, and more. Cells become less sensitive to insulin, predisposing to diabetes. Atherosclerosis and other vascular damage commonly occur in early diabetics, even those with normal cholesterol levels. Inactivity increases CHD risk by mechanisms other than an abnormal HDL/LDL ratio, including constriction of blood vessels. The vascular channels in a well-trained or fit cardiovascular system are broader. Smoking damages blood vessel walls, including coronary arteries. Hypertension puts increased stress on specific areas in blood vessel walls; it is often a result of excessive stimulation by the sympathetic nervous system. The underlying CAUSES of these problems are not disrupted HDL/LDL numbers. But the body's innate methods of dealing with them may RESULT in higher LDL and lower HDL.

Studies indicate that people who had suffered heart attacks had a lower HDL cholesterol primarily because they were older, fatter, had higher blood pressure, and smoked more than those who had not had a heart attack. Some studies did not find that HDL cholesterol was a major predictor or risk factor for CHD or, at best, was of marginal value for risk prediction. The researchers often admitted that the difference could as well have been due to other risk factors like stress or lack of exercise.

Theoretically, LDL cholesterol should have the strongest relationship to risk of CHD and should be a better predictor than total or HDL cholesterol. But it is not. Some studies found that total cholesterol, not LDL cholesterol, had a stronger relationship to risk of CHD. Others indicated there was a greater risk of heart attack if LDL cholesterol was low than if it was high. One report showed the predictive power of LDL cholesterol was statistically insignificant. An interesting study indicated that LDL was predictive for CHD only for men between ages thirty-five and forty-nine and only for women between ages forty and forty-four. A review of the studies leads to the conclusion that LDL cholesterol is not centrally or causally important; it does not have the strongest or most consistent relationship to risk for CHD. In fact, the endorsement of LDL cholesterol as a risk factor by the National Cholesterol Education Program is "loaded with misquotations and even false statements."

Many people with low HDL ("good") cholesterol have no CHD. Data eventually appeared that indicated a low HDL cholesterol level may not be so bad as long as enough of it is wrapped in a protein called apolipoprotein A-1 (apo A-1). Apolipoprotein B (apo B) was dubbed "bad" and thought to be a better predictor of cardiovascular risk than LDL. Yet, screening people for CHD by measuring apo B alone or with apo A-1 is "too poor to discriminate between recommending drug therapy or lifestyle change for some and not others." Not helpful.

Then some people were found to have small LDL cholesterol particles and others to have large LDLs. The smaller the LDLs, the greater the risk of CHD. Low-fat diets reduce LDL more in people with small particles than those with bigger particles. The smaller LDL particles are more easily oxidized (made rancid and toxic). However, people with larger LDL molecules tend to have abnormal levels of other blood fats. So, it is difficult if not impossible to determine if particle size is an independent risk factor.

A high level of lipoprotein(a) (Lp(a)), a group of varied particles in the blood closely related to LDL, was thought to increase risk of CHD and stroke. But not all studies found this, and it is not known if lowering high Lp(a) levels will prevent CHD. Diet does not seem to affect Lp(a) levels. However, a high Lp(a)—above 30 milligrams— may not be harmful if the LDL level is normal. In others words, it is not an independent risk factor. Some studies found no evidence of an association between Lp(a) and risk of future CHD. A study of people over 100 years of age found that 25 percent of this group had high Lp(a) serum levels even though they never had atherosclerosis- related diseases. Most of these folks also had low HDL levels and relatively high triglyceride levels, which together are considered to be strong risk factors for CHD. *Trans* fatty acids (altered, detrimental fats found in margarines, shortenings, partially hydrogenated veg- etable oils, fried foods) may raise Lp(a) levels. Saturated fats from whole, natural foods lower Lp(a). A large study suggested that ele- vated Lp(a) may be the result of coronary artery damage rather than a cause.

Since data show that people who live long may have "risk" fac- tors for CHD yet manage to live that long without atherosclerotic problems like heart attacks, the conclusion must be that the numbers (HDL, LDL, Lp(a), etc.) change according to the individual's needs as he/she ages, the degree of toxic offence, and need for repair, and do not indicate risk for heart attacks.

Oxidation of low-density lipoprotein is thought to be involved in CHD somehow. This means the problem with LDL cholesterol is not so much its presence or its quantity in the blood, but that it is easily oxidized or made rancid. This rancidity may contribute to tissue in- sult or injury. What causes LDL to become oxidized? For one thing, consumption of damaged or altered fats in the diet introduces to the tissues unstable, rancid, unnatural fats that can be poisonous and harmful. Most commercial vegetable oils fit this category. So do partially hydrogenated fats—containing trans fatty acids (found in most processed foods)—which have been shown to significantly increase the risk of CHD. Foods that are stored too long, stale, degraded, denatured, deteriorating, chopped, ground, mixed, or prepared also contain increased amounts of oxidized cholesterol molecules and fats as well as decreased amounts of antioxidants and other nutrients that prevent excessive or premature oxidation. Refined sugars increase oxidation damage, cross-link proteins, inhibit immune functions, and interfere with the transport of vitamin C complex (essential to the integrity of blood vessel walls). Deficiencies of nutrients that protect LDL—including the antioxidant portions of nutrient complexes as well as their more functional parts—contribute to the problem. Deficits of the vitamins A, B, C, and E complexes have been implicated as well as minerals like calcium, magnesium, potassium, selenium, etc., many phytochemicals, and fatty acids.

In multiple studies, "dietary cholesterol was not a predictor of plasma total or LDL cholesterol levels." But a high intake of calories, primarily from nonfoods containing little or no nutritional value, has been associated with elevated cholesterol levels. A high intake of refined carbohydrates (refined sugars and flours, etc.), for example, can result in elevated insulin levels, which may increase cholesterol levels. A diet low in refined carbohydrates lowers elevated total and LDL cholesterol.[3]

Low Cholesterol Levels

Numerous reports and studies indicate that **low** levels of blood cholesterol are associated with increased rates of depression, mood disorders, aggressive or disorganized behavior, violence, stroke, and suicide. These are just the adverse effects known at this time. Adequate serum cholesterol is needed for the proper function of the brain including its serotonin receptors. Serotonin is called one of the "feel good" biochemicals. People with chronically low cholesterol levels often show reduced serotonin levels. Cholesterol serves as precursor for almost all steroid hormones such as pregnenolone, estrogen, progesterone, testosterone, DHEA, and cortisol—all of which can affect mood and behavior.

Cholesterol levels below 150 are potentially harmful. A good portion of the population already takes drugs to force their cholesterol levels lower, and half the population is targeted for administration of statin drugs in the future. Such a widespread practice of forcing cholesterol levels lower through severe diets or toxic drugs for supposed reductions in heart disease risk raises some serious questions. In fact, a study spanning about 20 years showed that long-term low cholesterol increases the risk of death in the elderly. The earlier people experience lowered cholesterol concentrations, the greater the risk of death. Researchers are now beginning to question whether there is "scientific justification for attempts to lower cholesterol" to concentrations below 180 mg/dl in elderly people. Elderly people are at higher risk for heart attacks, but lowering their cholesterol levels—especially too low—actually increases their risk for death.

Removing as many dietary sources of fat and cholesterol as is possible may, for a time, cause the body to mobilize, reabsorb, and digest stored excess fats. But after six to twelve weeks or so, the excess fats will be gone and problems can begin to develop. Lowered sexual activity, impotence, dry skin, fatigue, loss of energy and motivation, premature aging and wrinkling, nervousness, irritability, depression, and other consequences are not unusual. It is also not unusual for blood concentrations of cholesterol to stay where they were or to go even higher. During the last two decades, the death rate from heart disease has dropped. During the same period, the nation's fat intake dropped a mere 6 percent. Perhaps emergency medical treatment is one reason the death rate has dropped, though CHD is still the number one killer. Whatever the reason(s) for the lowered death rate, "it isn't the low-fat diet, and it isn't reduced intake of dietary cholesterol."[4]

To be continued... in **Part 2.**

"Cholesterol, Fats, and Heart Attacks, Part 1" was originally published in *Nutrition News and Views,* July/Aug 2003, 7(4).

[1] D Williams, *Alternatives,* Aug 1999, 8(2):12; *Acres USA,* Dec 1996, 26(12):5; M Enig, *Wise Traditions,* Summer 2001, 2(2):46; J Mercola, *Townsend Lttr D&P,* Aug/Sept 1998, 181/182:20–1; T Cowan, *Wise Traditions,* Winter 2001, 2(4):46–

7; John R Lee MD Medical Lttr, June 2001:1–3; R Murray, Hlth Freedom News, Oct 1994, 13(10):44–7; U Ravnskov, Acres USA, Nov 2002, 32(11):30–2; W Douglass, Second Opinion, Nov 1994, 4(11):4.

2 U Ravnskov, The Cholesterol Myths (Washington: New Trends Pub., 2000) 15–133; J Mercola, Townsend Lttr D&P, Aug/Sept 1998, 181/182:20–21; U Ranskov, Acres USA, Nov 2002, 32(11):30–2; Lancet, 7 Aug 1993, 342(8867):355; M Balick, P Cox, HerbalGram, Summer 1997, 40:54; Amer J Pub Hlth, Aug 1998, 88(8):1202–5; John R Lee MD Med Lttr, June 2001:1–3; K Herron, et al., J Amer Coll Nutr, June 2002, 21(3):250–8; U Ravnskov, Lancet, 1 Dec 2001, 358(9296):1907 & 5 Nov 1994, 344(8932):1297; S Laidlaw, HealthLine, Mar 1999, 18(3):2; A Rijnsburger, et al., Lancet, 18 Oct 1997, 350:11; I Schatz, et al., Lancet, 4 Aug 2001, 358(9279):351–5; S Fallon, M Enig, Hlth Freedom News, Apr/May 1996, 15(2):24–7; M Mogadam, et al., Arch Intern Med, Aug 1990, 150:1645–8; W Callaway, Nutr Today, Sept/Oct 1994, 29(5):32–6; W Verschuren, et al., JAMA, 12 Jul 1995, 274(2):131–6; Hlth Freedom News, May 1995, 14(3):23–4; Health, Apr 1999, 13(3):25; F Sacks, Lancet, 29 Oct 1994, 344(8931):1182–6; Tufts Univ Hlth & Nutr Lttr, Jan 2003, 20(11):3; D McNamara, J Amer Coll Nutr, Dec 1997, 16(6):530–4; J Marshall, et al., Am J Clin Nutr, May 1998, 67(5):934–9; W Douglass, Sec Opinion, Dec 1994, 4(12):1–3; J Schmid, Health, Jul/Aug 1998, 12(5):95–101; S Rogers, Total Wellness, Jul 2001:1; UC Berkeley Wellness Lttr, Feb 1998, 14(5):4.

3 H Loomis, Chiropractic J, Jul 1997, 11(10):40–1; John R Lee MD Med Lttr, June 2001:1–7; UC Berkeley Wellness Lttr, Dec 1997, 14(3):7 & Oct 2001, 18(1):7; Nutr Act Hlthlttr, Jan/Feb 1993:4; Hlth, Mar/Apr 1995, 9(2):13–14; E Barnathan, JAMA, 10 Nov 1993, 270(18):2224–5; P Ridker, et al., JAMA, 10 Nov 1993, 270(18):2195–9; G Baggio, et al., FASEB J, Apr 1998, 12(6):433–7; PPNF Hlth J, Spring 1997, 21(1):14; Nutr Week, 4 Oct 1996, 26(38):7; J Bishop, Wall St J, 18 Nov 1992: B1; S Aldridge, Lancet, 12 Oct 1996, 348(9033):1021; S Ramsay, Lancet, 9 Sept 2000, 356(9233):917; G Warnick, et al., Lancet, 25 May 2002, 359(9320):1863–4; A Bostom, et al., JAMA, 21 Aug 1996, 276(7):544–8; C Gardner, et al., JAMA, 18 Sept 1996, 276(11):875–81; J Coresh, et al., JAMA, 18 Sept 1996, 276(11):914–15; G Walldius, et al., Lancet, 15 Dec 2001, 358(9298):2026–33; B Lamarche, et al., JAMA, 24 June 1998, 279(24):1955–61; N Wald, Lancet, 8 Jan 1994, 343(8889):75–9; S Ehara, et al., Circulation, 2002, 103:1955–60; M Muldoon, et al., Arch Med, 27 Mar 1995, 155:615–22; U Erasmus, Fats that Heal; Fats that Kill (Burnaby: Alive, 1993), 332–4; U Ravnskov, The Cholesterol Myths: 78–93; B Millen, et al., J Clin Epidem, 1996, 49(6):657–63; Herbs Hlth, Mar/Apr 2001, 6(1):9.

4 T Partonen, Br J Psychiatry, 1999, 175:259–62; J Brunner, et al., Pharmacopsychiatry, 2002, 35:1–5; B Golumb, et al., J Psychiatric Res, 2000, 34:301–9; L Ellison, et al., Epidem, 2001, 12:168–72; J Mercola, Townsend Lttr D&P, Aug/Sept 1999, 193/194:167 & June 2000, 203:146, cit Psychosomatic Med 2000: 62; R Rozzini, et al., BMJ, 18 May 1996, 312(7091):1298–9; J Behav Med, 1 Dec 2000, 23:519–29; PPNF Hlth J, Spring 1997, 21(1):14; Lancet, 2001, 358:351–5; H Loomis, Chiro J, Aug 1997, 11(11):40; HlthFacts, Feb 2003, 28(2):5–6.

Cholesterol, Fats, and Heart Attacks, Part 2

One-fifth of Americans (about 59 million) have coronary heart disease (CHD). Many factors contribute to the problem, but attention has been focused on cholesterol and dietary fats. Part 1 of this article showed that neither cholesterol levels nor various lipoproteins (such as HDL, LDL) in the blood appear to be directly related to heart attacks; neither does cholesterol consumed in the diet. What about other types of fats?[1]

Triglycerides

Triglycerides are the most prevalent fats in food and in the blood. They are essential for good health; tissues rely on them for energy. Currently the normal blood range for triglycerides is between 100 to 200 milliliters per deciliter. The cutoff of 200 was selected for ease of memory—it is the same cutoff number used for cholesterol. The blood level of triglycerides depends on and is influenced by many factors including ingestion of food. The level after a meal can rise several hundred percent higher than that of the fasting state. Up to 12 hours must pass before the level returns to "normal" (base). Anyone who eats three times a day, snacks, and has an occasional glass of wine will have values that are "too high" most of the time. Since triglyceride levels change throughout the day (rising and falling), a blood measurement is meaningless unless the person has been fasting for the previous 12 hours. Normal fasting levels are highly variable among individuals, and analysis of blood levels is highly inaccurate. If a lab analysis finds 200 mg/dl, the true level may be anything between 100 and 300 mg/dl. For a more reliable measure of the normal level, the average of at least three measurements made at three different occasions (each preceded by 12 hours of fasting) needs to be calculated.

Some studies seem to incriminate high triglyceride levels as a CHD risk factor. One study found the risk of having a first heart attack was more than twice as high in those with the highest triglyceride levels as in those with the lowest levels. The Physicians' Health Study reported that, for every 100-point rise in triglycerides, the risk of a heart attack climbed 40 percent. Another study found that high triglycerides alone increased the risk of heart attack nearly threefold. It has been suggested that the ratio of triglycerides to HDL is a stronger predictor of heart attack than the LDL/HDL ratio. Yet researchers admit there "still isn't proof that high triglycerides **cause** heart disease."

Overweight people have higher levels than thin people. Smokers have more than nonsmokers. Diabetics have higher levels than nondiabetics. People who lead a sedentary lifestyle have more than physically active people. Persons under stress have higher amounts than people at ease. Overweight, smoking, inactive, stressed, and diabetic people have more heart attacks than others. Is this due to higher triglyceride levels or are the elevated triglycerides a result of factors that contribute to CHD? It is easy to blame and medically treat triglycerides (with drugs such as niacin or Lopid). Weight loss, smoking cessation, exercise, and "blood sugar control" are more difficult but the best ways to lower triglycerides. These actions also lower heart attack rates. But a direct relationship between lower triglycerides and fewer heart attacks has not been shown.

"Going overboard on carbohydrates," specifically refined carbohydrates, can raise triglycerides. High triglycerides are "clearly related to high insulin levels" brought on by confounding the pancreas with insults of refined carbohydrates—foods stripped of nutrients and other components that assist the body in handling sugars and starches properly. Refined carbohydrates not only lack nutrients, they deplete bodily nutrients. Unless the calories are immediately used for energy, the excess are stored as triglycerides. A person with elevated triglycerides who dramatically reduces consumption of refined carbohydrates will almost always lower his or her levels. A diet of whole, natural foods and supportive supplements (to compensate for years of nonfood abuse) usually aids triglyceride levels fairly quickly. Triglycerides do not cause CHD; they reflect underlying factors that may do so.

Extra carbohydrate or fat calories are converted to fat (triglycerides) by the liver. Overweight persons with high insulin levels have higher fat formation rates than do lean persons with normal insulin levels. However, people with either high insulin levels OR normal insulin levels placed on a low-fat, high-carbohydrate diet with more than half of the carbohydrates in the form of **simple (refined) sugars** have high fat formation and increased triglyceride concentrations. Meaning? "The low-fat, high-carbohydrate diet often recommended as a substitution for high-fat, low-carbohydrate diets may not be the best possible choice…especially when most of the carbohydrate is in the form of simple sugars" as this can induce fat formation and insulin resistance. Carbohydrate-containing whole foods are not harmful; refined, ravaged, robbed, ruined carbohydrates are the culprits.[2]

Dietary Fats

For several decades, reducing dietary fat intake has been promoted to decrease CHD risk. Yet despite all the studies, experience, and time, it is still a controversial issue whether dietary fat *per se* is an independent risk factor for CHD. Based on the premise that it "may" influence CHD, Americans are advised to reduce total and saturated fats to 30 percent and 10 percent (respectively) of daily calories while increasing their intake of complex carbohydrates.

When people decrease dietary fats they increase—not proteins (usually associated with fats)—but carbohydrates, mostly REFINED carbohydrates. These raise insulin levels, lower HDL cholesterol, and elevate triglycerides (as much as 70 percent). "Research suggests that very low fat diets may trigger changes that increase risks of heart disease." Specifically, "high-carbohydrate, low-fat diets produce metabolic effects which would tend to increase the risk of heart disease…." So, "replacing saturated fat with carbohydrates will not reduce coronary heart disease risk."

A 1997 study challenged the notion that higher dietary fat *ipso facto* means increased CHD risk. A diet containing 42 percent fat did not cause any deterioration in heart rate, blood pressure, serum lipids, or exercise performance. Other research has had similar findings. "Several lines of evidence" indicate that the **types** of fats in the diet are more important in determining CHD risk than the total amount of fat. However, the "optimal mixture of different fatty acids" remains unsettled. "It has been increasingly recognized that the widely promoted low-fat concept is too simplistic and not compatible with available scientific data." Yet due to the vigorous campaign against fats, the belief that "all fat is bad" is strongly imbedded and widespread.

In the prestigious journal *Science*, Gary Taubes exposed the fact that, despite fifty years of mainstream research and hundreds of millions of research dollars, it has not been proved that eating a low-fat diet will help people live longer. Some people may benefit from lowering their consumption of some types of fat, he writes, but for people who eat a "reasonable" diet rich in whole foods such as fruits and vegetables, there is a question as to whether there are benefits sufficiently large to warrant concern. "It also questions whether all Americans will benefit from a low-fat diet." Decades of low-fat recommendations have "led many Americans to replace saturated fats with carbohydrates, not unsaturated fats." The data reveal that low-fat diets do not prevent deaths, and even if they seem to delay death, the effect is "marginal at best."[3]

Saturated Fats

Saturated fatty acids (SFAs) are often implicated in CHD risk, particularly long-chain SFAs. The claim is that saturated fats increase serum cholesterol levels and "harmful" LDL cholesterol, supposedly linking saturated fats, cholesterol, and CHD. SFAs are thought to raise blood cholesterol levels more than foods high in cholesterol. But the scientific basis for these assumptions is being questioned due to "large-scale misinterpretation and misrepresentation of the data." Foods containing high SFAs include animal fats like red meats, lard, dairy products (whole milk, cheese, ice cream, butter, etc.), chocolate, palm oil, palm kernel oil, and coconut oil. Hydrogenated vegetable oils could be included in this list, but they contain unnatural trans fatty acids, a different story.

One reason saturated fat is supposed to be bad is its high amount of calories. But other fats, including vegetables oils, are just as loaded with calories. Saturated fats like butter and coconut oil actually contain slightly lower levels of calories than polyunsaturated oils. Another reason for the saturated fat attack is that it is easily converted by the liver into cholesterol. Eating saturated fats is assumed to raise blood cholesterol levels, which is believed to increase risk of CHD. But this has not been shown to be true, and neither saturated fat nor cholesterol has been shown to cause CHD. Besides, the liver converts other substances such as carbohydrates and other fats into cholesterol as well.

In one trial, a group of participants consumed a high–polyunsaturated, low–saturated fat diet, and the controls continued their high–saturated fat, low–polyunsaturated fat diet. The low-SFA group experienced eight deaths from heart attacks. The high-SFA group experienced no heart attack deaths. In numerous studies (such as the Roseto, Irish Brothers, and Malhotra studies), it was found that those with the "wrong" fat composition in their diet (high saturated fat) were having far fewer heart attack deaths than people on high–polyunsaturated, low–saturated fat diets. A 1998 study in India found that the prevalence of CHD and "coronary risk factors" was higher in people with BOTH low- AND high–saturated fat intake. The Fulani (a Nigerian seminomadic pastoral group) consume a diet rich in saturated fats, do not use tobacco, are lean, and have an active lifestyle. "Despite a diet high in saturated fat," the Fulani have low risks for CHD.

Stearic acid, an SFA, has been exonerated from upping plasma cholesterol concentrations because the body readily converts it to a "neutral" monounsaturated fatty acid, oleic acid. Some scientists still consider stearic acid "thrombogenic" (causing blood clots). Other scientists say stearic acid may lower total and LDL cholesterol. Palm oil, a saturated fat previously viewed as virtual artery poison, also received a "bad rap." It does not raise blood cholesterol levels. Another misaligned fat, coconut oil, contains a type of saturated fat with "unique health properties," is no longer associated with arterial plaque buildup (atherosclerosis) and does not increase risk of heart disease. Ironically, over the past twenty-five years, coconut oil and palm oil in foods have been replaced by partially hydrogenated vegetable oils containing trans fatty acids—fats conclusively shown to be dangerous.

Findings from a large study "do not support the strong association between intake of saturated fat and risk of coronary heart disease.... Although a direct association between saturated fat intake and risk of coronary disease has been reported in several studies, those findings may have been confounded by fibre [fiber] intake.... Benefits of reducing intakes of saturated fat and cholesterol are likely

75

to be modest unless accompanied by an increased consumption of foods rich in fibre." A diet of whole, natural foods—unrefined and unaltered—would fit the bill. Biochemist Michael Gurr wrote "that whatever causes CHD, it is not primarily a high intake of SFAs. By the same token, major changes in SFA consumption are unlikely to lead to major benefits from CHD reduction." Research shows either a nonsignificant association between heart attacks and saturated fat intake or no association at all. Dr. William Castelli, director of the famous Framingham study, stated that "the more saturated fat one ate, the more cholesterol one ate, the more calories one ate, the lower the person's serum cholesterol." He conceded that "the people who ate the most cholesterol, ate the most saturated fat, ate the most calories, weighed the least, and were the most physically active."

Because saturated fats have no double carbon bonds—weak links that are easily broken—they are much more stable than polyunsaturated oils. Exposure to light, oxygen, and heat (normal cooking temperatures) does not result in an immediate or appreciable degree of oxidation—they are not easily altered or made rancid. These qualities make them preferential for use with food.

Still, Americans may consume excessive amounts of SFAs because they get inadequate amounts of other needed fatty acids. One reason for the imbalance is the manner in which meat animals are now raised. Ruminant animals, like cattle, are fed large amounts of grain, which is not natural for them. Their meat has four to six times more total fat and twice as much saturated fat than meat from totally grass-fed cattle. Milk from grass-fed cows contains up to five times (500 percent) more conjugated linoleic acid (CLA) than milk from standard, grain-fed cows. Milk from grass-fed animals contains more beneficial fats including well over twice as much omega-3 fatty acids as milk from grain-fed cattle. The same is true for chickens, turkeys, and eggs; free-range poultry have more beneficial fatty acids than commercially raised poultry. Free-range chickens have 21 percent less total fat, 30 percent less saturated fat, and 28 percent fewer calories. The meat has 50 percent more vitamin A and 100 percent more omega-3s. Free-range eggs contain almost twenty times more omega-3 fatty acids than supermarket eggs. People who traditionally and historically have eaten generous amounts of animal food were, in essence, eating different food. Is saturated fat "bad"? No. It is the distortions, deficiencies, and denaturing that takes its toll. Food raised in compliance with Nature's directions never contributes to CHD or any other problem.[4]

Trans Fatty Acids

Trans fatty acids (TFAs) have been conclusively linked with CHD. They raise LDL cholesterol levels, lower HDL cholesterol levels, increase lipoprotein(a) levels, raise triglyceride levels, **impair the ability of blood vessels to dilate**, and **interfere with essential fatty acids metabolism**. People consuming the most trans fats have a 50 to 66 percent higher risk of CHD than those consuming the least amount. A 14-year study of over 80,000 nurses showed that the women who consumed the largest amounts of trans fats had a 53 percent increased risk of suffering a heart attack than those at the low end of trans fat consumption. Total fat intake had little effect on the heart attack rate. Women with the largest consumption of total fat (46 percent of calories) had no greater risk of heart attack than those with the lowest consumption of total fat (29 percent).

TFAs occur in fats that have been "chemically altered by manufacturing processes" to hold a solid shape (as margarine) or thicken foods (as peanut butter). TFAs are formed when mono- or polyunsaturated oils are heated to high temperatures, changing the fatty acid molecules. Heat converts normal unsaturated fatty acids with their natural *cis* structure into saturated fatty acids with a toxic, unnatural *trans* structure. Hydrogen is added to make the oils more solid and stable. Hydrogenation gives margarine, shortening, and pudding a creamy consistency, and prolongs the shelf life of cookies, chips, crackers, cakes, popcorn, chocolate, and other foods that contain these semisolid oils. Partially hydrogenated oils stay solid at room temperature and do not become rancid as quickly as unaltered oils. Rancidity causes unpleasant tastes, so for salability, trans fats are preferred.

TFAs are found in thousands of processed foods including cakes, cookies, French fries, corn chips, doughnuts, Danish pastries, biscuits, white bread, pies, stick margarine, soft margarine, and vegetable shortening. Margarine may be the most common source in the

United States. But partially hydrogenated oils and shortenings added to processed foods contribute more to the overall consumption of trans fats than margarine. About 40 percent of ALL foods available in grocery stores contain TFAs. They can easily be avoided by eating unrefined, whole, unprocessed, nonfried, unaltered foods.

A study involving several European countries found that, in every country where there was low consumption of margarine and high consumption of **either olive oil or butter**, there was a very low incidence of death from heart disease. Belgium and Norway both consumed the same amount of margarine—a whopping 25 pounds per person per year. But Belgium consumes twice as much butter and twice as much olive oil as Norway. Norway is among the top countries experiencing deaths from CHD and Belgium is sixth from the bottom. This indicates that butter or olive oil (or both) is protective against the atherogenic effects of margarine. Spain and France are two countries with the lowest death rates from heart disease. People in Spain eat lots of olive oil but little butter; France has one of the highest butter-consumption rates. Consumption of olive oil or butter does not seem to matter. Avoidance of margarine and other trans fats makes the difference.

But, some may argue, trans fatty acids occur "naturally" in meat and dairy products. True, but "not all trans fatty acids may be harmful." The trans fats in meat do "not seem to increase the risk of myocardial infarction [heart attack]," **unlike** the trans fats in human-made partly hydrogenated fats. The former are natural; the latter are not. The body knows the difference. The artificial trans fatty acids created by technology are foreign to the body and cannot be used in a productive manner. Foods containing trans fats are promoted as containing "no cholesterol," yet they raise plasma cholesterol levels far more than natural saturated fat– and cholesterol-containing foods like butter, meat, or whole milk. Hydrogenated oils "may be the most destructive food additive currently in common use." They are used for deep-frying in fast-food restaurants. The fast-food industry switched from beef tallow to these trans-infested vegetable oils due to consumer demand for a "healthier" fat. They got just the opposite! Many researchers believe that TFAs have a greater influence on the development of CHD than any other dietary fat. Studies clearly show that trans fatty acids can contribute to atherosclerosis and heart disease—not because they are fats, but because they are altered, unnatural fats. "These are probably the most toxic fats ever known." CHD has multiple causes of both known and unknown origin. Trans fats are obviously one of them.[5]

Polyunsaturated Fats

The best known polyunsaturated fatty acids (PUFAs) are omega-6 fatty acids (arachidonic, linoleic, gamma[y]-linolenic) and omega-3 fatty acids (eicosapentaenoic [EPA], docosahexaenoic [DHA], alpha[a]-linolenic [ALA]). Polyunsaturated fats (such as corn, sunflower, safflower, and soy oils) seem to lower total blood cholesterol levels, particularly LDL (so-called bad) cholesterol. They were hailed as the most healthful oils to replace saturated fats. However, researchers have found that PUFAs also lower HDL (so-called good) cholesterol. Since a low HDL level is believed to be a risk factor for CHD, people are now nudged to use monounsaturated fats (such as olive or canola oils) since they leave HDL intact. Polyunsaturated fats evidently harm the lining of blood vessel walls (endothelial damage) that leads to atherosclerosis and CHD. Correlations have been found between PUFAs in the diet and adipose (body) fat, serum fats, and plaques in arteries.

Linoleic acid, an omega-6 and major PUFA, is the most abundant fatty acid in aortic plaque. The fat in plaques is derived from plasma LDL (vehicles that deliver fats to cells) in which there is more linoleic acid combined to cholesterol than any other fatty acid. The consumption of polyunsaturated fatty acids has steadily increased over the past fifty years or so. Now the long-term safety of diets rich in the omega-6 form is being questioned. But a recent study in Israel did not find a risk association of CHD with linoleic acid stored in bodily tissues. Yet the researchers said this is "not conclusive evidence for its safety." Other studies have been just as vague and inconclusive, whereas some find clear risks.

Linoleic acid is an essential fatty acid—it must be supplied by foods on a regular basis. Are people consuming too much polyunsaturated fats or not obtaining the correct ratio with other fatty acids? Omega-6 fatty acids like linoleic acid must be balanced with omega-3 fatty acids, for example. This concept of fatty acid ratios in the diet **alone** being the cause of problems is "overly simple." Research shows that high PUFA intake along with low antioxidant intake (from fruits and vegetables) is associated with increased CHD risk. Antioxidant portions of food complexes protect PUFAs and other fats from premature rancidity or breakdown. But this is not the entire solution either.

The processing methods for vegetable oils and the disturbed fatty acid levels in commercially raised animals have created biochemical disruptions and imbalances that contribute to CHD and other problems. PUFAs are unstable, lacking hydrogen atoms needed for stability, and are highly susceptible to "oxidative modification"—rancidity. The more unsaturated it is, the more unstable it is. In hundreds of studies, processed vegetable oils have been shown to harm the immune system and produce cancer in animals. In humans, excess consumption is associated with inflammatory and allergic diseases as well as cancers. Most fats in foods sold at supermarkets are processed PUFAs including cooking oils, salad dressings, baked goods, snack foods, and other items. Many are trans fats, polyunsaturated fats "spoiled by industrial hydrogenation."

When commercially extracted, the polyunsaturated oils are subjected to very high temperatures that promote rancidity and the formation of harmful breakdown products. They are then deodorized to remove the smell of rancidity. In other words, people consume large amounts of imbalanced, decomposed, putrid fats that are highly toxic. They consume inadequate amounts of fresh, natural (untampered-with) whole foods containing healthful PUFAs—vegetables, fruit, whole grains, raw nuts and seeds, legumes, fish, meat, eggs, and whole dairy products. Researchers recommend more polyunsaturated fats in the diet, "principally from cereals and vegetables," not from commercial oils and processed foods. Whole foods and their natural fatty components do not cause heart attacks. It is the altered, denatured, disrupted, fats that contribute to degeneration and disease.[6]

Omega-3 Fatty Acids

Sufficient amounts of omega-3 fatty acids are grossly lacking in the typical American diet. People in the United States consume far more omega-6 fatty acids than the omega-3 group. Many randomized trials have demonstrated that dietary or supplemental intake of omega-3 fatty acids significantly helps to lower risk of CHD, reduce risk of fatal heart attacks, prevent second heart attacks, prevent sudden death, and lower overall mortality. Data suggests that omega-3s may have an antiarrhythmic effect (assisting regular heart rhythm), may decrease heart rate variability, modestly reduce blood pressure, reduce elevated triglyceride levels (up to 30 percent), and improve arterial compliance (flexibility) and endothelial (blood vessel lining) function. The "synergistic effects" of omega-6 and omega-3 fatty acids are inversely related to CHD prevalence.

Recent research indicates that inflammation occurs with CHD. Inflammation is the body's method of attempting repair. People given supplementary omega-3 fatty acids from fish have less inflammation and stronger arterial plaques (thicker with more fibrous caps) than controls. Since plaques are "patches" to support and reinforce weak or damaged areas in blood vessel walls, the stronger the "patches," the less need for continued inflammation and repair. Omega-3s reduce the rate of growth of atherosclerostic plaque because they help reduce the need for more "patches" and enhance plaque stability. The "vulnerability of plaque to rupture is the primary determinant of acute thrombosis-mediated cardiovascular events."

ALA (alpha-linolenic acid) is an essential fatty acid of the omega-3 group. ALA is precursor to the long-chain omega-3s EPA (eicosapentaenoic acid) and DHA (docosahexaenoic acid). Ingestion of ALA or EPA and DHA from foods or supplements elicits benefits. However, there is controversy regarding the extent of conversion of ALA into EPA and DHA when foods contain ALA and little or no EPA and DHA. Fish is one of the best sources of the end products EPA and DHA. ALA, primarily found in vegetable-source foods, must be converted to EPA and DHA by desaturase enzymes in the body. Trans fatty acids can or do inhibit the various enzyme conversions. Avoidance of manufactured trans fats would no doubt improve conversion capacity. Rich ALA sources include leafy greens (purslane also contains a small amount of EPA), flaxseeds, several types of nuts, canola and soy oils, avocado oil, and more. Plants grown in the wild or organically tend to contain more omega-3s than those grown conventionally. Meat, poultry, eggs, and dairy products from animals raised entirely on pasture or free-range contain far more omega-3s than commercial types.

Supplemental fish sources of omega-3s might bring a quicker response, but vegetable sources "work" just as well though they may take a little longer for measurable results, perhaps six to twelve months. It takes time to incorporate nutrients into the biochemistry. Scientific studies do not usually last for months. Supplemental intake of isolated EPA and DHA may cause adverse reactions including gastrointestinal upset, clinical bleeding, a fishy aftertaste, worsening blood sugar metabolism, and a rise in LDL cholesterol. Whole food sources make more sense. Fish oil, such as cod liver oil, would seem to be an ideal supplement, but the "use of fish oil cannot be recommended in general" because it can contain significant levels of methylmercury (mercury), polychlorinated biphenyls (PCBs), dioxins, and other environmental contaminants. Processes that remove the contaminants often remove most of the nutrients too. But molecular separation (skimming off low–molecular weight components that hold the contaminants) leaves high–molecular weight components and concentrated nutrients like vitamin A complex and fatty acids such as the omega-3s.[7]

Monounsaturated Fatty Acids

The most common monounsaturated fatty acid (MUFA) is oleic acid. The best-known source of oleic acid is olive oil. Yet oils from foods such as avocado and nuts (like hazelnuts) have higher levels of oleic acid than olive oil. Canola oil—a bioengineered low–erucic acid rapeseed oil—has become a popular source of oleic acid. And high-oleic varieties of sunflower and safflower oils are appearing. A new type of palm oil is being grown that yields high oleic oil. Peanut oil is a good source. But all these vegetable-source oils must be non-hydrogenated to be of value. Many animal fats including tallow, lard, butter, chicken fat, eggs, and human milk are also high in oleic acid.

Oleic acid evidently inhibits oxidation (rancidity) of LDL cholesterol. This is one reason why olive oil and a Mediterranean diet are credited with preventing CHD. However, there are many sources of oleic acid, some oils containing more than olive oil. There is at least one other compound in olive oil (and another substance in whole olives) that may have protective effects on the cardiovascular system by a different mechanism. Olive oil has been researched far more than other MUFA-containing oils and foods, which may also contain their own unique nutrients or other components that are just as or more protective.

MUFAs are much more stable and resistant to oxidation (rancidity) than PUFAs. The oils are less likely to be partially hydrogenated or subjected to high heats. Heat is less damaging to MUFAs than it is to PUFAs. So MUFAs are less likely to cause biochemical disturbances and more likely to retain nutrients. **Extra virgin** olive oil contains the highest concentrations of flavonoids, nutrients supportive to the integrity of the blood vessel walls. It should also be remembered that a Mediterranean-type diet characteristically provides plenty of whole grains, fresh vegetables, fruits, and legumes—all supplying nutrients supportive to cardiovascular health—with little or no altered, denatured, toxic fats such as hydrogenated oils. While MUFAs may be beneficial to the cardiovascular system, it may also be the absence of manufactured, toxic fats and limited consumption of refined, overly processed, contaminated foods that contribute to the healthful reputation of a Mediterranean diet.

People in Italy, Greece, and Spain who consume huge amounts of olive oil enjoy better health and longevity than Americans. Inhabitants of Sardinia, where cancer and CHD are rare, drink olive oil by the glassful. Not only are their traditional diets composed of whole, natural, locally raised foods, but the olive oil they consume is different. Their oils are greenish, opaque, and thick, whereas the olive oil in the United States is yellow and clear, an indication that nutrients have been filtered out to give the oil a "pure" appearance. Humans should not tamper with Nature's creations; all fresh, complete, unchanged foods support health, repair, and balance.[8]

*To be concluded…*in **Part 3.**

"Cholesterol, Fats, and Heart Attacks, Part 2" was originally published in *Nutrition News and Views*, Sept/Oct 2003, 7(5).

[1] AHA's Heart & Stroke Statistical Update, *BMJ*, 1999, 318:79.

[2] T Farrell, *Veg Times*, Feb 2003, 306:67–72; *Hlth News*, 11 May 1998, 4(6):6; *Circulation*, 21 Oct 1997, 96:2250–2525 & 24 Mar 1998, 97:1027–36; *Nutr Act Hlthlttr*, Mar 1997, 24(2):6; M Miller, et al., *J Amer Coll Cardiol*, May 1998, 31(6):1252–7; C Hamilton, *Clin Prls News*, Oct 1998, 8(10):164; J Mercola, *Townsend Lttr D&P,* Aug/Sept 1998, 181/182:20 & Jun 1998, 179:28; *Women's Hlth Lttr*, Sept 1997, 6(9):6; J Schwarz, et al., *Am J Clin Nutr*, Jan 2003, 77(1):43–50; U Ravnskov, *The Cholesterol Myths* (Washington: New Trends, 2000), 94–5.

[3] *Circulation*, 1998, 98:935–39; J Mercola, *Townsend Lttr D&P*, Nov 1998, 184:52; J Jeppesen, et al., *Am J CLin Nutr*, Apr 1997, 65(4):1027–33; W Willett, *Proc Soc Exp Bio Med*, 2000:187–90; J Leddy, et al., *Med Sci Sports Exerc*, 1996, 29:17–25; S Dickerman, *Compl Med for Physician*, Aug 1997, 2(7):52–3; F Hu, et al., *NEJM*, 1997, 337:1491–99; F Hu, et al., *J Amer Coll Nutr*, Feb 2001, 20(1):5–19; *Wise Traditions*, Summer 2001, 2(2):8; G Taubes, *Science*, 3 Aug 2001, 293(5531):803–4; U Ravnskov, *Acres USA*, Nov 2002, 32(11):30–32.

[4] W Conner, *Am J Clin Nutr*, Aug 1996, 64(2):253–4; K Borie, *Eating Well*, Winter 2003, 1(3):10; P Kris-Etherton, et al., *Nutrition Today*, May/June 1993, 28(3):30–8; W Martin, *Townsend Lttr D&P*, July 1998:111–12; R Singh, et al., *J Amer Coll Nutr*, Aug 1998, 17(4):342–50; R Glew, et al., *Am J Clin Nutr*, Dec 2001, 74(6):730–6; *Eating Well*, Spring 2003, 1(4):10; A Ascherio, et al., *BMJ*, 13 Jul 1996, 313(7049):84–90; J Robinson, *Why Grassfed is Best* (Vashon: Washon Isl Press, 2000), 11–42; B Fife, *Healing Miracles of Coconut Oil* (Col Springs: HealthWise, 2001), 41–65; M Enig, *Know Your Fats* (Silver Spring: Bethesda, 2000), 76–7.

[5] F Hu, et al., *NEJM*, 20 Nov 1997, 337(21):1491–99; M Katan, et al., *Canadian J Cardiol*, Oct 1995, 11(suppl):36G–38G; A Ascherio, et al., *Circulation*, Jan 1994, 89(1):94–101; R Mensink, et al., May 2003, 77(5):1146–55; L Gatto, et al., *Am J Clin Nutr*, May 2003, 77(5):1119–24; T Farrell, *Veg Times*, Feb 2002, 306:67–72; A Lichtenstein, et al., *NEJM*, 24 Jun 1999, 340(25):1933–40; *Amer Health*, Jun 1994, 13(5):90–1; W Willett, et al., *Lancet*, 6 Mar 1993, 341(8845):581–5; *Nutr Today*, Jan/Feb 2003, 38(1):4; W Douglass, *Sec Opinion*, Feb 1998, 8(2):2–3; M Goldstein, *Lancet*, 29 Apr 1995, 345(8957):1108; *UC Berkeley Wellness Lttr*, Apr 2002, 18(7):1–2; L Litin, F Sacks, *NEJM*, 23 Dec 1993, 329(26):1969–70; B Fife, *The Healing Miracles of Coconut Oil* (Colorado Springs: HealthWise, 2001), 48–51; *Nutr Week*, 19 May 2003, 33(10):1.

[6] *UC Berkeley Wellness Lttr*, Jan 1995, 4(4):8; E Somer, *Nutr Report*, Nov 1993, 2(11):82; M Crawford, *Lancet*, 28 Jan 1995, 345(8944):256; A Truswell, *Lancet*, 28 Jan 1995, 345(8944):257; J Kark, et al., *Am J Clin Nutr*, Apr 2003, 77(4):796–802; E Vos, *Am J Clin Nutr*, Feb 2003, 77(2):521–2; *Wise Traditions*, Spring 2003, 4(1):48–9; U Ravnskov, *Acres USA*, Nov 2002, 32(11):30–2; C Felton, et al., *Lancet,*, 29 Oct 1994, 344(8931):1195–6; TL Roberts, et al., *British Heart J*, Dec 1993, 70(6):524–9; M Enig, *Know Your Fats* (Silver Spring: Bethesda, 2000), 37–8, 104–6.

[7] HC Bucher, et al., *AM J Med*, March 2002, 112:298–304; E Ross, *Nutr in Clin Care*, May/June 2000, 3(3):132–8; RN Lemaitre, et al., *Am J Clin Nutr*, 2003,

77:319–25; F Hu, et al., *JAMA*, 10 Apr 2002, 287(14):1815–21; F Thies, et al., *Lancet*, 8 Feb 2003, 361:477–85; R Greenfield, *Alt Med Alert*, Apr 2003, 6(4):47–8; W Douglass, *Real Hlth*, Jan 2003, 2(9):7–8; *NEJM*, 2002, 346(15):1113–18; R Lemaitre, et al., *Am J Clin Nutr*, Feb 2003, 77(2):319–25; W Harris, *Am J Clin Nutr*, Feb 2003, 77(2):279–80; M Zoler, *Fam Prac News*, 15 Jan 2003, 6; J O'Keefe, W Harris, *Am J Cardiol*, 15 May 2000, 85:1239–41; A Simopoulos, et al., *J Am Col Nutr*, 1992, 11:374–82; *UC Berkeley Wellness Lttr*, Feb 2002, 18(5):8; C Hamilton, *Clin Pearls News*, Jul 2000, 10(7):129; O Ezaki, et al., *J Nutr Sci Vitaminol*, 1999, 45(6):759–72; E Schmidt, et al., *Public Hlth Nutr*, 2000, 3(1):91–8; PM Kris-Etherton, et al., *Arterioscler Thromb Vasc Biol*, Feb 2003, 23:151–2; *Women's Hlth in Prim Care*, Jan 2003, 6(1):25–6; M Enig, *Know Your Fats* (Silver Spring: Bethesda, 2000), 28, 245.

8 A Gaby, *Townsend Lttr D&P*, June 1998, 179:37; *Eating Well*, Mar/Apr 1997, 7(4):55; F Visioli, G Galli, *Nutr Rev*, 1998, 56:142–7; M Enig, *Know Your Fats* (Silver Spring: Bethesda, 2000), 36–7; F Kliment, *Acid Alkaline Balance Diet* (Chicago: Contemporary Books, 2002), 29–30.

Cholesterol, Fats, and Heart Attacks, Part 3

Most people associate heart attacks with "deposits of cholesterol" that "clog" the opening in blood vessels (lumen of the coronary arteries). Yet the plaques lining the inside of blood vessels contain other substances such as white blood cells, calcium, platelets, and more. Cholesterol is not even the principle component of arterial plaque. Protein, mostly as scar tissue, is more abundant. Besides, 50 to 60 percent of people who had heart attacks did not have high cholesterol levels.

Actually, many heart attacks occur in people who have calcification of the middle layer of the coronary arteries, not excessive plaquing inside the vessel walls. This calcification or hardening of arterial walls—**arterio**sclerosis—can work its way to the outside of the artery. It occurs to reinforce weakness in or injury to the arterial wall, sort of like plaster or cement pumped in to strengthen a debilitating structure. Further deterioration of or stress on blood vessel walls or loss of elasticity (due to weakness or replacement of elastic tissue with a harder calcium substance) can lead to an aneurysm—a sudden rupture or "blow out"—resulting in hemorrhage and possibly death.

Atherosclerosis, though, has to do with plaque buildup on the inner wall of the coronary arteries, almost always at "stress points" or areas that receive the most pressure or mechanical tension. These areas are first to deteriorate (develop lesions) if there is injury, insult, or gradual degeneration of blood vessel walls. It has been known since the nineteenth century that degeneration of blood vessel walls starts BEFORE plaques appear in the lesions. Cholesterol is one substance used to patch or repair damaged or fragile areas of arterial walls. Blood vessel walls are in trouble BEFORE cholesterol-containing plaques appear. Plaques are the means by which the body attempts to prevent leakage and death.

Platelets stick to each other and to damaged tissue wherever there is injury, "plugging up holes" in blood vessel walls, for example, and providing "glue" by which cholesterol and other patch materials can adhere to vessel walls and to each other. The resultant blood clot causes the arterial cells to release protein growth factors that attempt to stimulate growth of muscle cells within artery walls. A complex combination of scar tissue, cholesterol, platelets, calcium, triglycerides, and white blood cells is attracted to the site in order to try to repair injured or deteriorating areas. This mass of fibrous tissue causes the plaquing where it is reinforcing the arterial wall and attempting to heal tissues. The plaque grows inside the artery wall, becomes part of it. Because strong circular muscles in the wall prevent the plaque from expanding outward, it pushes inward where (if large enough) it will narrow the artery opening. The more damage, deterioration, or chronic stress in the affected area, the more the plaque may grow, causing the opening to narrow. With substantial narrowing, or more likely, with constriction or spasm of the coronary artery, blood flow to the heart is interrupted or stopped. A heart attack.

In response to arterial injury, more cholesterol is directed to the affected area for reinforcement and mending. "Cholesterol is one of the body's major repair substances." Since cell walls and organelle membranes contain a lot of polyunsaturated fatty acids that are more easily oxidized than cholesterol, the cholesterol becomes oxidized in the plaque to try preserving the inner cells. HDL cholesterol carries oxidized cholesterol back to the liver for disposal. LDL cholesterol delivers fresh cholesterol to the site. As one pathologist put it, cholesterol does not cause plaquing any more than white blood cells cause an abscess.

Recent research has explored the inflammation process in relation to CHD. Some feel CHD does not occur in the absence of inflammation. When there is damage or deterioration of arterial walls, the inflammatory response is a protective and proactive attempt by the body to strengthen and repair tissues. Due to continual stress or breakdown, chronic inflammation may develop in an area. The body's efforts cannot keep up with continuous assaults OR there is a lack of nutritional fuel to accomplish adequate repair and strengthening. C-reactive protein (CRP) is one marker of systemic inflammation; levels rise when cellular injury and/or bacterial accumulation (due to cellular damage) occur. CRP levels may be useful in indicating acute coronary syndromes. Chemical mediators called cytokines are also being monitored in CHD. They elicit important effects in the inflammatory response, such as giving rise to platelet aggregation and coagulation or spurring functions of various white blood cells.

Repeated cycles of insult, irritation, injury, repair attempts, and reinjury to blood vessel walls may occur. Without sufficient support from a strong, healthy immune system and without ample supplies of all nutrients needed for inflammatory functions and for the strength and integrity of tissues involved, plaques may rupture, prompting emergency clots to form in order to prevent arterial rupture. This may lead to a heart attack (myocardial infarction), or a heart attack may lead to formation of emergency clots. Or, biochemical imbalances or deficiencies in nerves or smooth muscle tissues of blood vessels may result in spasm (sudden contraction), cutting off blood flow to the heart. Or, with severe arterial weakness, an aneurysm (excessive dilation and rupture of a blood vessel, like a bubble and blowout in an old bicycle tire) will also naturally prompt a clotting response, or, even worse, a massive, rapid loss of blood. When arterial degeneration exists, heart attack prevention means: (1) the plaques or "patches" must be strong enough to protect the arterial lesion or weak area, and/or (2) the arterial walls must not reach a point of deterioration that is so severe that plaquing cannot keep up with degeneration, and/or (3) extensive plaquing that dangerously narrows blood vessel openings does not develop so that a spasm or constriction will obstruct blood flow. Nutrition may play a vital role.

The strength, integrity, proper elasticity, and relaxation of blood vessel walls are thus prime considerations. However, in even healthy people, some thickening or fatty streaks may be found where arteries branch or make a turn—areas subjected to the greatest amount of pressure from blood. If the person's blood vessels are healthy and robust, and—should there be some injury—the "patching" is strong enough, then excessive narrowing or severe constriction does not occur.[1]

Nutrition and CHD

Numerous researchers have been critical of the cholesterol/fat/ heart attack hypothesis. Dietary intervention trials with low-cholesterol, low-fat diets have failed to support the flawed premise. The hypothesis "was formulated and popularized before adequate evidence was collected to establish its efficacy...this evidence, to date, is still lacking." Incomplete and invalidated research "continues to be used as the ultimate basis for dietary recommendations." Studies have shown that dietary fat does not necessarily raise serum cholesterol levels, that serum cholesterol levels are not a principle cause of arterial plaquing, that atherosclerosis does not always lead to frank cardiac disease. Clinical manifestation of CHD is low compared with the prevalence of coronary plaquing. Death may occur with minimal atherosclerosis; extensive atherosclerosis may not become clinically apparent, let alone result in death. Major studies on therapies that lower cholesterol may show some decrease in cardiac mortality but not in total mortality, "even after applying questionable selection methods and statistical treatment exaggerating effects of drugs and diet." Epidemiologic studies are inconsistent. For example, it has been shown that the rate of CHD in Japan decreased 40 percent over the previous twenty-five years as total dietary fat doubled and saturated fat intake increased. Many populations consume a high amount of saturated fatty acids without increased incidence of CHD.

The cholesterol/fat/heart attack premise has "always been a hypothesis in search of verification." Although cardiologists understand and evidence proves CHD to be a multifactor process, the popular conception of CHD as the end result of fat and cholesterol accumulation still prevails. "The public is led, or misled, to believe that prevention is mostly a matter of cutting back on fat intake, whereas nutrition is assigned the singular role of instructing people to reduce saturated fat" or total dietary fat. The scientific literature, however, testifies that many nutrients and foods help to prevent and treat CHD, such as:

Vitamin C complex with its rutin and flavonoids intact is critical to the strength and integrity of blood vessel walls as well as to the maintenance of proper elasticity in the vasculature. Vitamin C complex is imperative to the production of collagen and all connective tissue (including the musculature of vascular walls) and to oxygen metabolism. Studies have linked low blood levels of vitamin C to increased risk for heart attack. In fact, 70 to 80 percent of patients with heart disease have very low levels of vitamin C in their blood. Low plasma concentrations of vitamin C predict the presence of "unstable coronary syndrome," but the extent of atherosclerosis does not. Stress quickly depletes tissue levels. A deficit results in increased susceptibility of arterial walls to weakness, tearing, and chronic inflammation.

The association of excessive homocysteine with CHD has renewed focus on the importance of the vitamin B complex. Deficiencies of vitamins B_6, B_{12}, and folate are related to the severity of the hardening or stiffness of arteries as well as the degree of plaque buildup. Other B vitamins are also essential in areas such as nerve function and thus to blood vessel constriction and dilation, heart muscle function, and more. A deficiency of vitamin B_1 (involved in the heart's production of energy) increases the chances of having a heart attack. Refined carbohydrates deplete B_1 stores in the body as well as other B vitamins and associated nutrients. Overcooking and overprocessing of foods depletes or obliterates B vitamins. Synthetic B_1 and B_2 added to enriched flours interferes with proper use of B_6.

Vitamin E complex, including its selenium component, is supportive to blood vessel pliancy and integrity, heart function and rhythm, and adequate oxygen transport. Among other uses, oxygenation of the blood can help neutralize toxic waste particles that injure the lining of blood vessels and the heart. This contributes to the body's ability to break down and eliminate injured cells and to generate new cells. The E complex is essential for cellular respiration, especially in cardiac muscle. It promotes relaxation and proper dilation of blood vessels. High intake of omega-6 fatty acids from refined vegetable oils can increase the body's requirements for vitamin E. Refining and bleaching of flour abolishes the vitamin E content of grains. Intake of vitamin E results in up to 40 percent fewer coronary events.

Adequate intake of various minerals and trace minerals, including magnesium, potassium, calcium, selenium, chromium, copper, zinc, and others, is important to protect blood vessels and cardiac muscle. A combination of magnesium deficiency and consumption of trans fatty acids can produce atherosclerosis. Supplemental magnesium can reduce the risk of angina, cardiac arrest, and death. It may help prevent coronary artery constriction as does potassium and other minerals. Copper deficiency can damage arteries and the heart. Copper and zinc help create healthy collagen. Selenium deficits have been linked to CHD and to fibrotic lesions in the heart. With the rest of the vitamin E complex, selenium may reduce or eliminate angina attacks.

Omega-3 fatty acids lower the incidence of CHD, as does consumption of any unrefined, unaltered fat and foods containing natural fats. Carotenes, vitamin A complex, lipoic acid, vitamin D complex, numerous phytochemicals (such as flavones, sterols, allicin, capsaicin, flavonoids like quercitin, etc.), coenzyme Q10 (and other coenzymes), glutathione, and various other amino acids all play roles in cardiovascular well-being and healing. Both vitamin A and D complexes have several functions including acting as catalysts for protein and mineral assimilation and supporting inflammation processes. Stress depletes vitamin A levels. Vitamin D helps prevent hypertension and protects against spasm. Various amino acids in bioavailable form are essential to the transport of fatty acids used by the heart to manufacture energy, to the strength and health of cardiac muscle and smooth muscle of blood vessels, to nerve conduction, to cholesterol and triglyceride levels, and more. Coenzyme Q10 (CoQ10) and associated coenzymes are involved in the production and transportation of energy in the heart. There is more CoQ10 in the heart than in any other organ. It is involved in inflammatory processes as well. Cholesterol-lowering drugs greatly increase the body's need for CoQ10. The antioxidant portions of nutritional complexes may perform as protectors—preventing damage from highly processed vegetable oils and prematurely oxidized bodily fats and cholesterol. Many other nutrients—or lack thereof—have been shown to influence cardiovascular health.

Consumption of refined sugars and starches, altered fats—particularly trans fatty acids—and any other food denatured or adulterated to the point of becoming a nonfood or antifood should be reduced or avoided.

Real foods and herbs such as onions, garlic, brassaca vegetables (broccoli, cabbage, etc.), green leafy vegetables, citrus fruits, berries, peppers, ginger, turmeric, ginkgo, legumes, apples, whole grains, and others too numerous to list here have been shown to protect tissues and help repair. Virtually ANY whole, natural food studied seems to show favorable effects. CHD is halved, for instance, in people with a high intake of fruits and vegetables. "The concept of synergy dictates that a broad spectrum" of nutrients serve best in preventing and ameliorating CHD. Whole foods are the best way to obtain the synergistic packages of nutrients and other ingredients embodied by Nature's balanced organization.

There is no question that the "real" nutrient content of diets—the intricate, codependent, intact network of interrelated nutrients and other natural components (known and unknown) found in whole foods—has declined during the last seventy or more years. Processed, denatured, refined nonfoods have replaced many nutrient-dense real foods. The content of minerals and other valuable substances have declined in soils. Manufactured, maimed, mutated, and embalmed fabrications are consumed with relish while real foods (like those containing the falsely accused fats) are neglected. Synthetic, isolated, inorganic, or fractionated "nutrients" in popular supplements are ingested in a vain attempt to make up for what is not consumed in wholesome, dynamic natural foods. Nutrient values in real foods will naturally vary. It is not the specific measurement of nutrients in foods that is most important. It is the synergistic power of the whole that packs the punch. Nutrients in whole foods work more efficiently and are needed in smaller quantities than synthetic imitations or separated portions.[2]

Cholesterol Balance

Thyroid imbalance, blood sugar disruption, liver stresses, genetic tendencies, overweight, eating disorders, and other factors may cause blood cholesterol elevations or decreases. Insult or injury to blood vessels or other tissues may also be causes. Unbalanced cholesterol or lipids are not diseases, but are signs that something is askew and the body is doing what it needs to do. What a person eats can also influence cholesterol levels, but not in the way usually publicized.

For example, the effect of any type of dietary fat on serum cholesterol levels depends on the original cholesterol levels, why the levels are where they are, and the fat itself. Almost ALL natural, unaltered fatty acids will help reduce elevated serum cholesterol levels and increase low levels. Although some studies seem to give an edge to monounsaturated fats (like olive, canola, or peanut oils) in lowering cholesterol, other studies do not. Highly polyunsaturated oils can "impressively" lower cholesterol. Diets rich in saturated fats can reduce total and LDL cholesterols. The key is the quality and form of the fat such as how the oil or fat is extracted and processed, whether or not it is rancid or contains toxins, if it has been altered. ANY fat the body does not recognize as a real and beneficial food will stress the liver and other areas, nudging extra production of cholesterol.

Low cholesterol values appear in both those who eat small amounts of animal fat and those who eat large amounts. Some studies try to prove that animal fats increase cholesterol levels by using a diet that lasts only a few weeks or even one day, but any sudden change in diet can cause temporary biochemical adjustments, not reflecting a food's actual effects. The best information comes from surveys conducted over long periods of time and during different seasons of the year. When this time-consuming, expensive method is used, researchers do not find any correlation between animal-fat intake and blood cholesterol.

People with elevated cholesterol levels "are likely to have a deficiency of essential fatty acids (EFAs)." Without sufficient EFAs, the liver may compensate by increasing cholesterol production. Correcting EFA insufficiency often helps lower elevated cholesterol levels. Most Americans are deficient in omega-3 fatty acids which, when supplied, reduce elevated cholesterol levels. Other fatty acids can be just as effective. Omega-6 fatty acids are consistently effective in lowering cholesterol. Gamma-linolenic acid (as in evening primrose or black currant seed oils) is often helpful.

Almost any whole, natural food can be favorable to cholesterol balance. Phytochemicals (such as phytosterols and saponins), fiber, legumes, whole grains, fruits, and vegetables can all lower total and LDL cholesterol. Garlic, ginger, cayenne, reishi, Indian myrrh tree, and psyllium have been studied for their beneficial effects on cholesterol balance. Liver-supporting foods and herbs often assist, such as dandelion, beets, radishes, milk thistle, burdock, Oregon grape root, and so on. Choline, inositol, and the rest of the B complex are needed by the liver to process cholesterol. Calcium, magnesium, potassium, and chromium have positive effects on cholesterol, LDL, HDL, and triglycerides. Blood levels of HDL cholesterol rise in step with blood levels of vitamin C; higher blood levels of vitamin C are associated with lower total and LDL cholesterol. Tocotrienols, components of vitamin E complex, have cholesterol-balancing effects. High vitamin

A intake correlates with higher plasma HDL and apolipoprotein A-1. "Weight loss is the most effective means" of balancing cholesterol, lipoprotein, and triglyceride values in overweight people. Regular exercise, especially if combined with a diet of natural, whole foods, will significantly assist cholesterol levels.

Whole, natural foods and herbs have benefits, not in direct action "against" cholesterol, but in their ability to empower the body's innate regulatory or management processes AND in their ability to reduce the need for aberrant cholesterol and lipid levels. Still, the principle of biochemical individuality must be considered. What will lower or balance cholesterol and lipids for one person may not do so for the next.[3]

Changes, Changes

Many foods have experienced status changes in relation to CHD and cholesterol levels. Eggs are one example. Egg yolks are among the most concentrated sources of cholesterol (about 215 mg each, whereas the recommended limit of cholesterol is 300 mg/day). People stringently restricted themselves to the occasional use of only egg whites. Now eggs, including yolks, are okay since they do not raise blood cholesterol levels. One major Harvard study found no association between consumption of one egg a day and greater risk for CHD or stroke. More eggs on a daily basis were not tested. The implication was that two eggs or more each day might be risky. But there is no evidence that eggs will cause any risk. "Feel free to eat all the eggs you want." The rediscovered egg is now praised for its health benefits as it contains nutrients such as folate, other B vitamins, "antioxidants," and unsaturated fats.

Nuts are a high-fat food, previously prohibited and now allowed. Many studies have shown positive associations between nut consumption and cardiovascular health and reduced CHD risk. Walnuts, pecans, hazelnuts, pistachios, almonds, macadamias, and other nuts have been studied. They are excellent sources of monounsaturated and polyunsaturated fatty acids; minerals like magnesium, potassium, and copper; fiber; vitamin E complex (nuts are one of the best sources); and protein. Total and LDL cholesterol elevations are reduced when nuts are part of the diet; HDL increases. Nuts do not contribute to obesity and can actually aid in weight loss programs. The public "should not be afraid of nuts." Eaten raw, nuts are not harmful, and "contain nutrients that make important contributions to a healthy diet."

Beef has been shunned by cholesterol-conscious people for years. But the various fatty acids in beef—especially from grass-fed cattle—do not pose the risk once feared. Most Americans identify replacing red meat with poultry and fish as an action that will help lower blood cholesterol levels. "However, elimination of beef from the diet may not be necessary" since both lean beef and lean chicken produce "significant decreases" in total and LDL cholesterol levels. No significant differences in total, LDL, or HDL cholesterol or in triglycerides were found when beef or chicken diets were consumed. Red meat is "a nutrient dense food" containing very important B vitamins, zinc, iron, and higher amounts of some trace minerals than poultry or fish.

For years people were warned to avoid shellfish due to its high cholesterol content. However, "this advice has been reversed." Even large quantities in the diet have "little or no effect" on blood cholesterol levels. No natural, unaltered food—including those rich in fats—will clog arteries or cause heart attacks or any other biochemical imbalance or health problem. Avocados, for example, are high in fat, rich in fiber, and are high in carotenes, vitamin C complex, E complex, and potassium. They are healthful, not harmful, as are any natural, intact, untampered-with foods.

Volunteers in a cardiovascular-rehabilitation program for more than a year were placed on an elimination and rotation diet. The diet eliminated all refined, processed, manufactured, and fried foods. At each meal, one or two types of food "in their natural state" were eaten, and unlimited quantities were allowed. There was a significant lowering of blood pressure and serum lipids and triglycerides. Body mass was lowered, HDL cholesterol was increased, glucose and insulin levels normalized. Fats are not the problem. Depleted, massacred, mangled, denatured, damaged, bungled nonfoods stand guilty.

For the past ninety years (during which time CHD rates were rising), the amount of fat in the American diet has been fairly constant at 35 to 40 percent of calories. The amount of fat in the diet is not a problem. Some traditional diets (Eskimo, Native American, African Maasai, etc.) contained 60 to 80 percent of calories as fat with virtually no incidence of heart disease. However, the **quality** or **form** of the fats IS an issue. Stable, nutrient-dense animal fats (butter, meats, eggs, seafood, etc.) and other whole, fat-rich intact foods (nuts, seeds, whole grains, avocados, olives, coconuts, etc.) have been replaced by refined, processed, often rancid vegetable oils; by stripped, depleted grains and refined sugars; and by other disassembled, depreciated, adulterated, perverted concoctions that are nutritionally impoverished, high in imbalanced components or toxic by-products; and devoid of the delicate synergy Nature places in all natural foods. Nonfoods and reformed foods lack the nutrients needed for a healthy cardiovascular system, cause imbalances that predispose to CHD, and provide toxins or breed harmful chemical descendants that harm or weaken cardiovascular tissues and functions.[4]

Not So Sweet

The work of numerous investigators has shown that **refined** carbohydrates elevate blood levels of cholesterol and triglycerides regardless of intake of various types of fats. Unrefined, whole food carbohydrate sources do not have this effect. Epidemiologic data demonstrate an "adverse impact" of sucrose ("white" sugar) and other refined carbohydrates on blood triglycerides and lipoproteins. Sadly, many studies show an association between carbohydrates and CHD risk without clarifying the difference between refined carbohydrates (stripped of most nutrients, cofactors, and fiber) and whole food carbohydrates. Whole foods have far more nutrients, intact fatty acids, and ingredients that aid proper blood sugar metabolism, fat metabolism, and biochemical utilization. They do not increase risk for CHD.

For instance, people on the island of St. Helena have a very high rate of CHD even though they do not smoke much, are physically active, and have a low-fat diet. However, the islanders do consume an annual average, per person, of 125 pounds of refined sugar. Some investigators are suggesting that carbohydrates should be given various ranks since research indicates that simple, refined carbohydrates increase risk while complex carbohydrates reduce risk. A diet high in refined carbohydrates can cause elevations in total and LDL cholesterol, triglycerides, glucose, insulin; a reduction in HDL; and insulin resistance.

Use of high-fructose corn syrup has increased tenfold since the 1970s. This refined sugar is selectively shunted to the liver without going through some intermediary breakdown steps to which other sugars are subjected. It greatly increases production of triglycerides, leads to insulin resistance, depresses enzymes used for "burning" fat, and increases enzymes that "burn" sugar rather than fat. Long-term ingestion of refined fructose causes increased fat formation, increased VLDL (so-called very bad) cholesterol, increased insulin and triglyceride blood levels, and decreased glucose tolerance. Overuse of fructose skews the metabolism toward fat storage (overweight) and increases risk for CHD. Fruit contains fructose, so the sugar is thought to be healthful, natural. But high-fructose corn syrup is a separated, refined, and processed sweetener that "is about the furthest thing from natural that one can imagine, let alone eat." Refined fructose now accounts for 9 percent of the average American's daily dietary intake and about 20 percent of the average child's diet. People are inundated with fructose-laden convenience foods, snacks, soda, and candy. Fructose is evidently a contributor to the rampant incidence of obesity, diabetes, and CHD.

Several studies directly linked milk to heart attacks. Theories pointing to unfermented milk protein, milk calcium, butterfat, saturated fat, and cholesterol were made, but none of them showed a clear connection. Then lactose and skim milk were found to have high associations with CHD. With pasteurization, milk sugar (lactose) is altered, changed from alpha-lactose to beta-lactose. The enzyme needed to properly digest and absorb lactose (lactase) is destroyed. Essentially, the lactose becomes a refined sugar, stripped of components needed for proper blood sugar metabolism, for handling by the liver, and for utilization by cells. Low-fat and skim milk, lacking the rich flavor and consistency of whole milk, are treated with chemical additives for body, texture, and mouthfeel. Dried milk—superheated with grossly denatured and "modified" protein—is added. Superheated and ultrapasteurized milk products are heated to 300°F, surpassing the critical temperature (191°F) above which milk becomes toxic or foreign to the body. Unaltered milk and fermented dairy products have cholesterol-lowering effects, increasing HDL and improving LDL/HDL ratios. Fermented products such as yogurt, acidophilus milk, and kefir increase gut bacterial contents, which ferment indigestible carbohydrates (like altered lactose), increase short-chain fatty acids in the intestines, and enhance bile-acid conjugation.

"The classic diet/heart hypothesis related to dietary fat and cholesterol is shown to be flawed in many respects. A much stronger dietary link to heart disease is consumption of sugars such as fructose, lactose, and sucrose"—REFINED carbohydrates.[5]

"Cholesterol, Fats, and Heart Attacks, Part 3" was originally published in *Nutrition News and Views*, Nov/Dec 2003, 7(6).

[1] S Rogers, *Total Wellness*, Jul 2001:1–2; R Dowdell, *Hlth Freedom News*, Sept 1992:25–28; N Rifai, P Ridker, *Curr Opin Lipidol*, 2002, 13:383–89; S Jee, et al., *JAMA*, 8 Dec 199, 282(22):2149–55; F Pashkow, *Cleveland Clin J Med*, Feb 1999, 66(2):75–77; S Fallon, M Enig, *Wise Traditions*, Spring 2001, 2(1):14–26; F Wassef, *Am J Nat Med*, Sept 1998, 5(7):12–17; B Fife, *The Healing Miracles of Coconut Oil* (Colorado Springs: Health Wise, 2001), 77–87; M Enig, *Know Your Fats* (Silver Spring: Bethesda, 2000), 77–80, F Kliment, *The Acid Alkaline Balance Diet* (Chicago: Contempory Books, 2002), 25–94.

[2] W Grant, *Am J Nat Med*, Nov 1998, 5(9):19–23; J Vita, et al., *J Am Coll Cardiol*, Apr 1998, 31(5):980–6; S MacRury, et al., *Scot Med J*, 1992, 37:49–52; F Kummerow, et al., *Am J Clin Nutr*, 1999, 70, cited in *Women's Hlth Lttr*, Jan 2001, 7(1):6; T Rissanen, et al., *Circulation*, 28 Nov 2000, 102:2677–9; C Gardner, *Coron Artery Dis*, 2001, 12:553–9; K Nelson, *Nutr Today*, May/Jun 1995, 30(3):114–22; S Fallon, M Enig, *Consum Res*, Jul 1996:15–19; A Simopoulos, *J Nutr*, 2001, 131:3065S–73S; R Nicolos, et al., *J Am Coll Nutr*, Oct 2001, 20(5):421S–7S; E Schaefer, *Am J Clin Nutr*, Feb 2002, 75(2):191–212; C Callaway, *J Am Coll Nutr*, Oct 1997, 16(5):491, Ab 79; A Gaby, *Townsend Lttr D&P*, Aug/Sept 2002, 229/230:26; J LaPuma, *Alt Med Alert*, Feb 2003, 6(2):22–3; H Gerstein, S Yusuf, *Lancet*, 6 Apr 1996, 347(9006):949–50; S Sternberg, *Sci News*, 25 May 1996, 149(21):324; F Hu, W Willett, *JAMA*, 27 Nov 2002, 288(20):2569–78; S Byrnes, *Hlthkprs*, Spr/Sum 2001, 3(1):13; L Linxue, et al., *Jpn Circ J*, Feb 1999, 63:73–8; F Wassef, *Am J Nat Med*, Sept 1998, 5(7):12–17.

[3] E Beauschesene-Rondeau, et al., *Am J Clin Nutr*, 2003, 77:587–93; *Nat Hlth*, Jul/Aug 1993:18; L Berglund, et al,. *Am J Clin Nutr*, 1999, 70:992–1000; *UC Berkeley Wellness Lttr*, Mar 1997, 13(6):1–2 & Feb 1998, 14(5):4 & Jan 2001, 17(4):5; A Adler, et al., *Am J Clin Nutr*, Jul 1997, 2(6):46–7; B Olson, et al., *J Nutr*, 1997,

127:1973–80; I Reid, et al., *Am J Med*, 2002, 112: 343–7; *Hlth News*, Jun 2002, 8(6):5; R Singh, et al., *Bio Tr El*, 1991, 30:59–64; J Hallfrisch, et al., *Am J Clin Nutr*, Jul 1994, 60(1):100–5; M Werbach, *Townsend Lttr D&P*, Feb/Mar 1998:180 & Apr 1998:156; S Lamon-Fava, et al., *Am J Clin Nutr*, Jan 1994, 59(1):32–41; L Lalonde, et al., *Prev Med*, 2002, 35:16–24; N Fuchs, *Women's Hlth*, Oct 2002, 7(10):1–3; A Fitzpatrick, *Intern J Integr Med*, Apr/May 2002, 4(2):8–20; D Nieman, *J Am Coll Nutr*, Aug 2002, 21 (4):344–50; M di Buono, et al., *J Nutr*, Aug 1999, 129:1545–8; *Herbs for Hlth*, Mar/Apr 2001, 6(1):9; U Ravnskov, *Cholesterol Myths* (Washington: New Trends, 2000), 96–112; L Seman, *Nutr Clin Care*, May/Jun 2000, 3(3):127–8; W Grant, *Am J Nat Med*, Nov 1998, 5(9):22; D McNamara, *Canad J Cardiol*, Oct 1995, G:113–26; *Hlthkprs*, 2003, 5(1):37.

[4] *Lancet*, 30 Mar 1991, 337(8744):787; *UC Berkeley Wellness Lttr*, Mar 1995, 11(6):6–7 & May 1998, 14(8):7; *Nutr Week*, 1 Dec 1995, 25(45):7 & 23 Apr 1999, 29(15):7; W Douglass, *Sec Opin*, Oct 2000, 10(10):6–7; R Rowan, *Sec Opin*, Mar 2003, 13(3):6–7; D Zambon, et al., *Ann Inter Med*, 4 Apr 2000, 132(7):538–46; A Gaby, *Townsend Lttr D&P*, Jan 2001, 210:132; M Abbey, et al., *Am J Clin Nutr*, 1994, 59:995–9; G Fraser, *Asia Pacif J Clin Nutr*, 2000, 9(sppl):528–32; K Edwards, *J Am Coll Nutr*, 1999, 18(3):229–32; W Morgan, *J Am Diet Assn*, 2000, 100:312–18; *Brit Med J*, 14 Nov 1998, 317(7169):1332–3; 1342–5; L Roberts, *Science*, 27 May 1988, 240:1149; L Scott et al, *Arch Inter Med*, 13 Jun 1994, 154(11): 1261-7; J Keenan et al, *Postgrad Med*, Oct 1995, 98(4): 113-26; D Hunninghake et al, *J Am Coll Nutr*, Jun 2000, 19(3):351–60; E Hiser, *Eating Well*, Mar/Apr 1992:94; *S Afric Med J*, Sept 1997, 87(9):1222; H Jiang, et al., *Am J Clin Nutr*, Feb 1995, 61(2):366–72; *Sci News*, 18 Nov 2000, 158(21):327; M Okita, et al., *Asia Pac J Clin Nutr*, 2000, 9(4):309–13; G Borok, et al., *Cardiovas J S Africa*, Apr 1995, 6(2):96–101.

[5] T Starc, et al., *Am J Clin Nutr*, 1998, 67:1147–54; C Vidon, et al., *Am J Clin Nutr*, May 2001, 73(5):878–84; L Van Horn, et al., *Nutr in Clin Care*, Nov/Dec 2001, 4(6):314–31; W Willett, *Soc Exp Biol Med*, 2000:187–90; K Hamilton, *Clin Prls News*, Jan 2002, 12(1):9; W Grant, *J Orthomolec Med*, 2nd Q 1998, 13(2), cited in *Townsend Lttr D&P*, Jul 1999, 192:25; G Reaven, *Am J Clin Nutr*, Nov 1997, 66(5):1293–6; J Jeppesen, et al., *Am J Clin Nutr*, Apr 1997, 65(4):1027–33; G Critser, *Fat Land* (NY: Houghton Mifflin, 2003), 136–40; R Rowan, *Sec Opin*, Mar 2003, 13(3):6; P St Onge, et al., *Am J Clin Nutr*, 2000, 56:843–9; W Grant, *Am J Nat Med*, Nov 1998, 5(9):19–23.

About the Author

Judith DeCava has worked independently, as well as an associate with physicians, nutritionists, and clinical psychologists for more than thirty-five years. She was chief consultant for R. Murray & Associates, Inc., of Florida and Missouri, being privileged to work with and learn from Richard P. Murray, DC, a brilliant biochemist, doctor, humanitarian, friend, and disciple of Dr. Royal Lee. After Dr. Murray's death, DeCava opened her own private practice as well as a research and consulting business in supplement formulation.

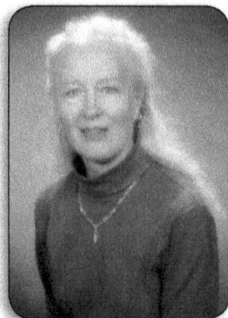

DeCava has been writing about health science since 1985 in articles, newsletters, and books. She was a regular contributor to the National Academy of Research Biochemists, Institute of Practical Biochemistry, and Biomedical Health Foundation. In her most well-known book, *The Real Truth about Vitamins and Antioxidants*, she describes the superiority of food complexes over isolated and synthetic chemical portions. She currently researches and writes her own newsletter, *Nutrition News and Views*, for health professionals, although it is frequently "shared" with the general public.

Her interest in nutrition and health began in her teens with a search to ascertain answers to her own health problems and a fascination with the influence and effects of foods and nutrition on living organisms and their well-being. At first, following the dictates of current scientific and general literature on health and nutrition, she tried isolated, synthetic, and inorganic supplements. After some years of working with physicians and becoming increasingly disappointed, confused, and puzzled with this line of "fake"—only barely effectual—therapy, she continued to hunt for answers, sure that there was some way, some pieces to the gigantic puzzle that would be more helpful. When, by accident, she obtained several newsletters written by Dr. Murray, the dawn began to break. A whole new world began to open with the revelation that whole foods and whole food nutritional complexes (supplements) were the factors for which people were starving, that deficiencies and imbalances were behind many ills and physical problems. Through some interesting circumstances and sheer determination, she eventually began to work with Dr. Murray and quickly became a consultant in his office for his patients. The lessons learned in practical biochemistry, anatomy, physiology, psychology, and plain old compassion went far beyond anything that could be absorbed in any of the formal courses she took or literature she read.

DeCava feels the more she learns, the more there is to learn. Her regard for Nature has always drawn her and elicited awe and reverence. Loss of health, in her view, frequently means the individual has lost touch with Nature, including loss of connection with his or her own body and Self. Rediscovering that connection with Nature and Self, including the use of Nature's foods and therapies, has become the goal of her own practice and the direction of her philosophy and writing.

Judith A. DeCava is a licensed nutrition counselor (Florida), a certified dietitian-nutritionist (New York), and a certified nutritional consultant (organizational). She is a professional member of the International Foundation for Nutrition and Health, the American Association of Nutritional Consultants, the Price-Pottenger Nutrition Foundation, and the American Botanical Council. She is an associate member of the American College of Nutrition and a member of the American Association for the Advancement of Science, the Weston A. Price Foundation, the American Herb Association, and the National Coalition Against the Misuse of Pesticides.

Resources

Websites/Blogs

www.seleneriverpress.com

The Dr. Royal Lee website, www.drroyallee.com

The SRP Self-Health Nutrition Blog, www.seleneriverpress.com/blog/

The Selene River Press Historical Archives, www.seleneriverpress.com/historical-archives/historical-archives-home

The Standard Process website, www.standardprocess.com/Our-Company/Home

The Weston A. Price Foundation, www.westonaprice.org/health-topics/royal-lee-dds-father-of-natural-vitamins/

Social Media

Like Selene River Press on Facebook

www.facebook.com/SeleneRiverPress

Follow Selene River Press on Twitter, Pinterest, and Google+

www.twitter.com/SeleneNutrition

Social Media ...

www.pinterest.com/SeleneRiverPress

plus.google.com/app/basic/+SeleneRiverPress/posts

Selene River Press Books and Products

Conversations in Nutrition by Dr. Royal Lee and John Courtney

Empty Harvest by Dr. Bernard Jensen and Mark Anderson

From Soil to Supplement: A Course in Food, Diet, and Nutrition, Taught by Dr. Royal Lee

Lectures of Dr. Royal Lee, Volume II presented by Dr. Royal Lee

Legendary Formulas of Dr. Royal Lee presented by Dr. Michael Dobbins

Put Your Money Where Your Mouth Is! Guide to Healthy Food Shopping by Stephanie Selene Anderson

SRP Self-Health Starter Kit™

The Foundations of Trophotherapy, Book One of the Selene River Press Foundations of Trophotherapy eBook Series

The Real Truth About Vitamins and Antioxidants by Judith DeCava

The Triad: Dr. Royal Lee and the Immune System presented by Mark R. Anderson

Vaccination: Examining the Record by Judith DeCava

Vitamin News by Dr. Royal Lee

Why Your Doctor Offers Nutritional Supplements by Stephanie Selene Anderson

www.ingramcontent.com/pod-product-compliance
Lightning Source LLC
Chambersburg PA
CBHW062103270326
41931CB00013B/3188